Accession no.
36176304

616.
07
Rof

Nurses! Test Yourself
Pathophysiology

✔ KU-285-680

WITHDRAWN

Nurses! Test Yourself in ...

Titles published in this series:

Nurses! Test Yourself in Anatomy and Physiology
Katherine M. A. Rogers and William N. Scott

Nurses! Test Yourself in Pathophysiology
Katherine M. A. Rogers and William N. Scott

Nurses! Test Yourself in Essential Calculation Skills
Katherine M. A. Rogers and William N. Scott

Visit www.mcgraw-hill.co.uk/openup/testyourself for further information and sample chapters from other books in the series.

Nurses!
Test Yourself in
Pathophysiology

Katherine M. A. Rogers and
William N. Scott

LIS LIBRARY

Date 11/4/13   Fund q-aat

Order No 2389988

University of Chester

Open University Press

Open University Press
McGraw-Hill Education
McGraw-Hill House
Shoppenhangers Road
Maidenhead
Berkshire
England
SL6 2QL

email: enquiries@openup.co.uk
world wide web: www.openup.co.uk

and Two Penn Plaza, New York, NY 10121-2289, USA

First Published 2011

Copyright © Katherine M. A. Rogers and William N. Scott 2011

All rights reserved. Except for the quotation of short passages for the purposes of criticism and review, no part of this publication may be reproduced, stored in a retrieval system, or transmitted, in any form or by any means, electronic, mechanical, photocopying, recording or otherwise, without the prior written permission of the publisher or a licence from the Copyright Licensing Agency Limited. Details of such licences (for reprographic reproduction) may be obtained from the Copyright Licensing Agency Ltd of Saffron House, 6–10 Kirby Street, London, EC1N 8TS.

A catalogue record of this book is available from the British Library

ISBN-13: 978-0-33-524223-8
ISBN-10: 0-33-524223-5
eISBN: 978-0-33-524224-5

Library of Congress Cataloging-in-Publication Data
CIP data applied for

Illustrations by Gary Holmes
Typeset by RefineCatch Limited, Bungay, Suffolk
Printed in the UK by Bell & Bain Ltd, Glasgow.

Fictitious names of companies, products, people, characters and/or data that may be used herein (in case studies or in examples) are not intended to represent any real individual, company, product or event.

Mixed Sources
Product group from well-managed
forests and other controlled sources
www.fsc.org   Cert no. TT-COC-002769
© 1996 Forest Stewardship Council
FSC

The McGraw·Hill Companies

PRAISE FOR THIS BOOK

"This book provides extensive coverage of each of the human body systems. It relates pathophysiology to the clinical environment, relevant investigations and treatments for disease. A useful text for both newly qualified and student nurses."

Amy Hutchinson, Student Nurse, University of Ulster, UK

"This book contains a substantial bank of questions which will prove very useful to any enthusiastic student wishing to actively learn and revise pathophysiology. The simple structure and expanded answers provide effective feedback, adding value and support for learning. The book will be a useful partner to support many of the pathophysiology textbooks currently available. It should be included on recommended reading lists for students. It will also find a useful place in support of teaching and professional development."

Jim Jolly, Head of Academic Unit for Long Term Conditions,
School of Healthcare, University of Leeds, UK

Contents

Acknowledgements

We wish to thank Rachel Crookes, Claire Munce, Della Oliver and the rest of the team at McGraw Hill-OUP for all their help and support throughout the writing of this text. We would also like to acknowledge all the reviewers who read our manuscript and provided us with very useful feedback.

About the authors

Dr. Katherine Rogers and Dr. William Scott are lecturers in applied health sciences with the School of Nursing and Midwifery at Queen's University Belfast where they teach health science subjects, including anatomy, physiology, pathophysiology and pharmacology to both undergraduate and postgraduate students of nursing science. They are also External Examiners in these subjects in a number of Higher Education Institutions across the UK.

Using this book

INTRODUCTION

Welcome to *Nurses! Test Yourself in Pathophysiology*. We hope you will find this an invaluable tool throughout your pathophysiology course and beyond!

This book is designed to be used as a revision aid that you can use with your main textbook. Each chapter is designed for stand-alone revision, meaning that you don't have to read from the beginning to benefit from the book – you can dip in and out as you need to.

Every chapter begins with a brief introduction covering the main points of the topic and directing you to some useful resources. The chapter progresses providing you with different types of questions that help you test your knowledge of the area. These are:

- *Labelling Exercise*: identify the different elements on the diagram.
- *True or False*: identify if the statement is true or false.
- *Multiple Choice*: identify which of four answers is correct.
- *Fill in the Blanks*: fill in the blanks to complete the statement.
- *Match the Terms*: identify which term matches which statement.

The questions have been designed to be slightly more challenging in each section. Do not ignore a question type just because you are not tested in that way because the answer contains useful information that could easily be examined in an alternative question format. Answers are provided in each chapter with detailed explanations – this is to help you with revision but can also be used as a learning aid.

We have suggested some useful textbooks that may be used to support your recommended text, but be aware that they should not replace the core reading for your course.

A list of common abbreviations used throughout the book and a list of common prefixes, suffixes and word roots commonly used in pathophysiology are provided. At the back there is a glossary.

We hope that you enjoy using this book and that you find it a convenient and useful tool throughout your studies!

GUIDE TO TEXTBOOK RESOURCES

Nurses! Test Yourself in Anatomy and Physiology
Katherine M. A. Rogers and William N. Scott
Published by McGraw-Hill, 2011

Fluids and Electrolytes Made Incredibly Easy
William N. Scott
Published by Lippincott Williams & Wilkins, 2010

Ross and Wilson's Anatomy and Physiology in Health and Illness (11th edition)
Anne Waugh and Allison Grant
Published by Churchill Livingstone, Elsevier, 2010

Symptoms, Diagnosis and Treatment: A Guide for Pharmacists and Nurses
Paul Rutter
Published by Churchill Livingstone, Elsevier, 2005

List of abbreviations

These are common abbreviations used in the clinical setting and throughout this book.

ABG	arterial blood gas	CVA	cerebrovascular accident (or stroke)
ACE	angiotensin-converting enzyme	CVD	cardiovascular disease
ACS	acute coronary syndrome	CVS	chorionic villus sampling
ADH	antidiuretic hormone (or vasopressin)	DEXA	dual energy X-ray absorptiometry
AIDS	acquired immune deficiency syndrome	DI	diabetes insipidus
		DKA	diabetic ketoacidosis
ALL	acute lymphocytic leukaemia	DM	diabetes mellitus
		DRE	digital rectal examination
AML	acute myeloid leukaemia	DVT	deep vein thrombosis
ASD	autistic spectrum disorders	ECG	electrocardiogram
AST	aspartate aminotransferase	EEG	electroencephalogram
BP	blood pressure	EMG	electromyography
BUN	blood urea nitrogen	ERCP	endoscopic retrograde cholangio-pancreatography
CAD	coronary artery disease		
CF	cystic fibrosis	ESWL	extracorporeal shock wave lithotripsy
CK	creatinine kinase		
CKD	chronic kidney disease (end-stage renal disease)	FH	familial hypercholesterolaemia
		GCS	Glasgow Coma Scale
CLL	chronic lymphocytic leukaemia	GFR	glomerular filtration rate
		GI	gastrointestinal
CML	chronic myeloid leukaemia	GP	general practitioner
CO_2	carbon dioxide	GTN	glyceryl trinitrate
COPD	chronic obstructive pulmonary disorders (or diseases)	HDL	high-density lipoprotein
		HDU	high dependency unit
CRF	chronic renal failure	HIV	human immunodeficiency virus
CSF	cerebrospinal fluid		
CT	computerized tomography	HNPCC	hereditary non-polyposis colorectal cancer
CTS	carpal tunnel syndrome		

HPV	human papilloma virus	PD	Parkinson's disease
HRT	hormone replacement therapy	PEFR	peak expiratory flow rate
HSV	herpes simplex virus	PID	pelvic inflammatory disease
ICP	intracranial pressure		
ICU	intensive care unit	PKU	phenylketonuria
IDDM	insulin dependent diabetes mellitus	PPI	proton-pump inhibitor
		PSA	prostate-specific antigen
IV	intravenous		
IVP	intravenous pyelogram	RBC	red blood cell (or erythrocyte)
IVU	intravenous urogram		
LAD	lactate dehydrogenase	RIRS	retrograde intrarenal surgery
LDL	low-density lipoprotein		
LP	lumbar puncture (or spinal tap)	SAH	subarachnoid haemorrhage
		SCLC	small-cell lung cancer
MI	myocardial infarction (or heart attack)	SOB	shortness of breath
		STEMI	ST-elevation myocardial infarction
mM	millimolar		
mmol/L	millimoles per litre	STI	sexually transmitted infection
MRI	magnetic resonance imaging		
Non-STEMI	non-ST-elevation myocardial infarction	TIA	transient ischaemic attack (or 'mini-stroke')
NSAID	non-steroidal anti-inflammatory drug	TSH	thyroid-stimulating hormone
		UTI	urinary tract infection
NSCLC	non-small-cell lung cancer	UV	ultra-violet
O_2	oxygen	VTE	venous thromboembolism
PCNL	percutaneous nephrolithotomy	WBC	white blood cell (or leucocyte)

Directional terms

Abduct   move away from the midline of the body; the opposite of adduct

Adduct   movement towards the midline of the body; the opposite of abduct

Anterior   front-facing or ventral; opposite of posterior or dorsal

Contralateral on opposite side; opposite of ipsilateral

Distal   far away from point of origin; the opposite of proximal

Dorsal   to the back or posterior of; opposite of ventral or anterior

Inferior   lower or beneath; opposite to superior

Ipsilateral   on same side; opposite to contralateral

Lateral   referring to the side, away from the midline; opposite of medial

Medial   towards the middle; opposite of lateral

Posterior   back or dorsal; opposite of anterior or ventral

Proximal   nearest to the centre of the body; opposite of distal

Superior   above or higher; opposite of inferior

Ventral   referring to front or anterior; opposite of dorsal or posterior

The table below summarizes how these terms match up.

Direction	Opposite term
Abduct	Adduct
Anterior/ventral	Posterior/dorsal
Contralateral	Ipsilateral
Distal	Proximal
Inferior	Superior
Lateral	Medial

Common prefixes, suffixes and roots

Prefix/suffix/root	Definition	Example
a-/an-	deficiency, lack of	*anuria = decrease or absence of urine production*
-aemia	of the blood	*ischaemia = decreased blood supply*
angio-	vessel	*angiogenesis = growth of new vessels*
broncho-	bronchus	*bronchitis = inflammation of the bronchus*
card-	heart	*cardiology = study of the heart*
chole-	bile or gall bladder	*cholecystitis = inflammation of gall bladder*
cyto-	cell	*cytology = study of cells*
derm-	skin	*dermatology = study of the skin*
entero-	intestine	*enteritis = inflammation of the intestinal tract*
erythro-	red	*erthyropenia = deficiency of red blood cells*
gast-	stomach	*gastritis = inflammation of stomach lining*
-globin	protein	*haemoglobin = iron-containing protein in the blood*
haem-	blood	*haemocyte = a blood cell (especially red blood cell)*
hepat-	liver	*hepatitis = inflammation of the liver*
-hydr-	water	*rehydrate = replenish body fluids*
leuco-	white	*leucopenia = deficiency of white blood cells*
lymph-	lymph tissue/vessels	*lymphoedema = fluid retention in lymphatic system*
myo-	muscle	*myocardium = cardiac muscle*
nephr-	kidney	*nephritis = inflammation of the kidneys*
neuro-	nerve	*neurology = study of the nerves*
-ology	study of	*histology = study of the tissues*
-ophth-	eye	*ophthalmology = study of the eyes*
osteo-	bone	*osteology = study of bones*
path-	disease	*pathology = study of disease*
pneumo-	air/lungs	*pneumonitis = inflammation of lung tissue*
-uria	urine	*haematuria = blood in the urine*
vaso-	vessel	*vasoconstriction = narrowing of vessels*

1 Introduction to pathophysiology

INTRODUCTION

The body is always striving to maintain an internal equilibrium called homeostasis, which is regulated by the brain and maintained by a number of positive and negative feedback mechanisms. Disease or illness may develop when homeostasis is disrupted. The study of pathophysiology (or pathobiology) considers the changes that occur in normal anatomy and physiology as a result of illness or disease.

Any cellular change or damage can affect the whole body. Injury, malnutrition or invasion by pathogens can all disrupt homeostasis. Cells check for such imbalances during replication and usually adapt successfully in response to such stresses. However, sometimes the dividing cell fails to detect unwanted changes and the resulting mutation may cause disease.

In the study of pathophysiology, we usually consider a number of factors: the causes of disease (aetiology), the changes to normal anatomy and physiology (pathophysiology), the signs and symptoms (clinical manifestations) of the disease or illness, along with diagnostic tests and treatments available.

This chapter examines changes in homeostasis and how this leads to illness or disease. To assess a patient's symptoms and be able to plan, deliver and evaluate their care, nurses need to understand how changes to normal anatomy and physiology can lead to the development of illness and disease.

Useful resources

Nurses! Test Yourself in Anatomy and Physiology

Chapter 1

Ross and Wilson's Anatomy and Physiology in Health and Illness (11th edition)

Chapters 1 and 3

TRUE OR FALSE?

Are the following statements true or false?

1 The division of somatic cells involves four stages.

2 During their lifetime, cells face constant challenges to their normal function.

3 There are two types of homeostatic feedback mechanisms.

4 Dysplasia describes a reduction in cell size.

5 Disease can develop when normal homeostasis cannot be sustained.

6 When assessing pain, remember the acronym PQRST.

7 Cancer is a condition that develops when cells die uncontrollably.

MULTIPLE CHOICE

Identify one correct answer for each of the following.

8 Homeostasis can be defined as:

a) functional changes caused by disease

b) an unbalanced state, out of equilibrium

c) a steady, dynamic state of equilibrium

d) the exaggeration of an original response

9 Which of the following regions of the brain is not involved in maintaining homeostasis?

a) pons

b) medulla oblongata

c) pituitary gland

d) reticular formation

10 How many components are there in a homeostatic feedback mechanism?

a) 6

b) 5

c) 4

d) 3

11 Which cellular adaptation describes an increase in the number of cells in response to an increased workload?

a) atrophy

b) hypertrophy

c) hyperplasia

d) metaplasia

12 The majority of solid cancerous tumours arise from:

a) glandular tissue

b) skin tissue

c) nervous tissue

d) epithelial tissue

13 The cellular transformation from a normal to a cancerous cell is called:

a) carcinogenesis

b) replication

c) mutation

d) necrosis

FILL IN THE BLANKS

Fill in the blanks in each statement using the options in this box.
Not all of them are required, so choose carefully!

chronic	remission
metastasize	illness
latent	metaplasia
organ	acute
carcinogenesis	contagious
tissue	referred
residual	aetiology
pathogenesis	

14 _____ describes the replacement of one adult cell with another.

15 The _____ of a disease can be intrinsic or extrinsic.

16 The development of a disease is called its _____.

17 Complete the stages in disease progression:

    i)   injury/exposure
    ii) _____ phase
    iii) prodromal period
    iv) _____ phase
    v)   _____
    vi) convalescence
    vii) recovery

18   The pain radiating along the left arm often reported by MI patients is called _____ pain.

19   A solid tumour is usually classified according to the _____ from which it originates.

20   Cancer cells can _____ away from their origin.

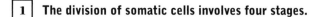

ANSWERS

 TRUE OR FALSE?

1 The division of somatic cells involves four stages.

Somatic cell division has two stages. The first stage is mitosis, when the nucleus and genetic material of the cell divide. In mitosis there are a number of different growth and synthesis phases. The second stage in cell reproduction is cytokinesis. At the beginning of this stage the cytoplasm divides; it ends when the new cell's contents divides into two new daughter cells (by convention, new cells are called daughter cells). In gametes (sex cells), cell division and reproduction occur by meiosis.

2 During their lifetime, cells face constant challenges to their normal function.

The normal functioning of the cell is constantly being challenged by stressors within the body and its external environment. The cell can normally adapt to such stressors and continue to function normally. However, sometimes the cell is unable to adapt to these challenges allowing stressors to induce changes to the body's state of health, causing disease or illness. When cells are stressed, they can undergo a number of changes: atrophy, hypertrophy, hyperplasia, metaplasia or dysplasia.

3 There are two types of homeostatic feedback mechanisms.

The two types of feedback mechanisms are: positive feedback and negative feedback. Positive feedback occurs when a stimulus triggers an enhanced response exaggerating the original event. Negative feedback mechanisms restore homeostasis by detecting and correcting changes to the normal homeostatic conditions in the body. There are fewer examples of positive feedback than negative feedback; examples include the platelet formation in the blood coagulation cascade (haemostasis) and oxytocin release during labour contractions in childbirth. Examples of negative feedback include secretion of insulin from the pancreas to reduce high blood sugar levels back to normal, control of body temperature by thermoreceptors in the hypothalamus (thermoregulation) and also the control of blood pressure and respiration rate.

4 Dysplasia describes a reduction in cell size.

Atrophy refers to a reduction in cell size. It can happen when cells are no longer used, are malnourished, have insufficient blood supply, lack of innervation or have insufficient hormonal stimulation. Dysplasia describes abnormal growth or development of tissues or cells, leading to a change in size, shape and appearance that is sometimes reversible but often precedes neoplastic (cancerous) changes.

5   **Disease can develop when normal homeostasis cannot be sustained.**

A disease will usually induce specific signs and symptoms that may require investigation. Disease develops following disruption of the body's normal homeostasis, while illness describes poor health caused by disease. Disease differs from illness because an individual may live a reasonably normal life and not be considered ill, despite having a disease. For example, an asthmatic person can live a normal life and not usually be considered ill because the body has adapted to the disease. However, the disease may make them more susceptible to certain illnesses such as respiratory infections or pneumonia.

6   **When assessing pain, remember the acronym PQRST.**

PQRST is a useful prompt to remember the questions to ask a patient when assessing pain.

P = *precipitation/palliation* – what causes the pain and what relieves it?
Q = *quality* – how could the pain be described, is it crushing, dull, sharp or stabbing?
R = *region/radiation* – where did the pain start and has it spread elsewhere?
S = *severity* – how bad is the pain, using a scale 0 = no pain to 10 = worst pain?
T = *timing* – when did the pain start and how long does it last?

7   **Cancer is a condition that develops when cells die uncontrollably.**

Cancer develops due to excessive and uncontrollable cell growth. A cancerous (or neoplastic) cell develops due to a mutation of a single cell which affects the control of normal function in the cell. The mutation allows the cell to grow and proliferate without the normal regulatory controls of cell growth and replication and it loses the ability to enter apoptosis (cell suicide). Initially the uncontrolled growth of the cancerous cells is localized but because they have lost the ability to perform apoptosis, the cells do not die and so the mass of proliferating cells begins to invade nearby tissue and may eventually metastasize to other areas of the body. Most cancers are solid tumours but malignancies can arise in the blood; these are called haematological cancers. Necrosis is an undesirable form of cell death usually caused by factors external to the cell, such as trauma, toxins or infection.

MULTIPLE CHOICE

Correct answers identified in bold italics

8 **Homeostasis can be defined as:**

a) functional changes caused by disease   b) an unbalanced state, out of equilibrium   *c) a steady, dynamic state of equilibrium*   d) the exaggeration of an original response

Homeostasis involves intricate and tightly controlled events that the body uses to preserve the stability of the internal environment of cells, tissues, organs and systems and hence helps keep the body in good health. Homeostasis helps to maintain the volume and temperature of body fluids so that the body exists in a favourable environment to remain healthy. It is controlled by the brain and is regulated by positive and negative feedback mechanisms. The hallmark of the ageing process is a decrease in the body's ability to maintain homoeostasis because the body becomes less able to adapt to stressors. For example, many individuals suffer from hypertension as they get older because the body becomes less able to adapt to changes in blood pressure.

9 **Which of the following regions of the brain is not involved in maintaining homeostasis?**

a) pons   b) medulla oblongata   c) pituitary gland
d) reticular formation

Three parts of the brain are involved in maintaining homeostasis in the body. They are the medulla oblongata in the brain stem, the pituitary gland and the reticular formation. The medulla oblongata controls a number of vital functions such as circulation and respiration. The pituitary gland controls the function of other glands and is involved in regulation of growth, maturation and reproduction. The reticular formation is a group of nerve cells that control certain vital reflexes such as cardiovascular function and respiration. The pons is located just above the medulla oblongata but is not involved in maintaining homeostasis. It houses a number of cranial nerves that are involved in interpreting sensory information.

10 **How many components are there in a homeostatic feedback mechanism?**

a) 6   b) 5   c) 4   *d) 3*

Every homeostatic feedback mechanism has three components: (1) a sensory mechanism – to detect deviations in the homeostatic equilibrium; (2) a control centre in the central nervous system – which regulates the body's response to the change; and (3) an effector mechanism – which receives responses from the CNS that help restore homeostatic equilibrium.

11 **Which cellular adaptation describes an increase in the number of cells in response to an increased workload?**

a) atrophy   b) hypertrophy   *c) hyperplasia*   d) metaplasia

Hyperplasia can also occur in response to hormonal stimulation or decrease in tissue mass. It differs from metaplasia, which describes replacement of cells rather than an increase in cell number. Hypertrophy describes an increase in cell size rather than increase in number of cells. Atrophy describes a destruction or shrinkage in cell size.

12 **The majority of solid cancerous tumours arise from:**

a) glandular tissue   b) skin tissue   c) nervous tissue
d) epithelial tissue

Any cancer derived from epithelial tissue is usually classified as a carcinoma. Cancers derived from glandular tissue are called adenocarcinomas. Tumours of the nervous tissue are termed gliomas. Tumours derived from supporting tissue such as muscle, bone and connective tissues, are called sarcomas. Lymphatic and immune system tumours are classified as lymphomas. Tumours of the white blood cells are leukaemias, while tumours of the pigment cells are called melanomas. Plasma cell tumours are classified as myelomas.

13 **The cellular transformation from a normal to a cancerous cell is called:**

a) carcinogenesis   b) replication   c) mutation   d) necrosis

There is no single cause that triggers carcinogenesis. It is likely to be induced by a number of triggers that interact together and that the cell is unable to defend against. These triggers can be genetic, lifestyle factors (smoking, diet, lack of exercise), hormonal, metabolic, viral, radiation, or chemical in nature. Carcinogenesis is a multi-stage process that involves a pre-clinical (latent) phase and a clinical phase. In some cancers, the latent phase can last for many years and in others it may be very short (weeks, months). The stages of carcinogenesis include:

I.   *initiation* – the spontaneous genetic mutation;
II.   *promotion* – confers a selective growth advantage that allows the abnormal cell to grow and proliferate;
III. *progression* – a series of additional mutations allow the mutated cell to continue to grow and evade apoptosis, by now the cells may not be distinguishable from the parent cell;
IV.   *metastatic spread* – the movement of cancerous cells away from their site of origin.

FILL IN THE BLANKS

14 *Metaplasia* **describes the replacement of one adult cell with another.**

The replacement cell is usually better able to withstand stresses and endure changes. Metaplasia is a type of cell adaptation that most often occurs in response to irritation or chronic inflammation.

15 **The** *aetiology* **of a disease can be intrinsic or extrinsic.**

The aetiology (or cause) of a disease can be influenced by the individual's biochemistry (intrinsic) or environmental (extrinsic) factors. Intrinsic biochemical factors are beyond an individual's control since they include factors such as age, gender and genetics. Extrinsic factors are influenced by lifestyle and the external environment. They can include stress, diet, drug use (prescribed and illicit), smoking, injury, bacteria or viral infections, exposure to chemical or radioactive agents, and exposure to extreme temperatures. Occasionally diseases arise that have no known aetiology, these are described as idiopathic.

16 **The development of a disease is called its** *pathogenesis.*

Most diseases have defined symptoms of progression that they will follow if left untreated. Some diseases are described as *self-limiting* because they resolve themselves without any interventions; other diseases will never resolve and are described as chronic. Patients with chronic diseases may experience periods of remission or exacerbation. During remission, symptoms improve or disappear while during exacerbation a patient may suffer increasing severity of symptoms. An example of a chronic condition that can undergo such periods is the inflammatory disease, rheumatoid arthritis.

17 **Complete the stages in disease progression:**

i)   injury/exposure
ii) *latent* phase
iii) prodromal period
iv) *acute* phase
v)   *remission*
vi) convalescence
vii) recovery

A disease progresses through a number of stages in the order described and is triggered by an injury or exposure to a pathogen. During the latent or incubation period, no signs or symptoms will be observed. During the prodromal period, mild signs and symptoms will be observed but are usually non-specific (such as headache, nausea, fever). In the acute phase the disease is at its peak, complications may arise in this phase. If the patient is still able to function in a reasonably normal manner, this phase may be called a subclinical acute phase. Remission is a second latent phase that occurs after the disease has reached its peak. It may be followed by a relapse into another acute phase. During convalescence the disease has passed and the patient progresses towards recovery. A patient is said to be recovered when there are no signs and symptoms of disease. At this stage the patient has generally returned to normal health.

18 **The pain radiating along the left arm often reported by MI patients is called *referred* pain.**

Referred (or reflective) pain describes pain experienced in part of the body at a distance from its area of origin. Referred pain is not completely understood but is thought to happen when nerve fibres from various regions or organs converge on the same levels of the spinal cord. The best-known example is pain experienced during a MI. Nerves from damaged cardiac tissue convey pain signals to spinal cord levels T1–T4 on the left side, which are the same levels that receive sensation from the left side of the chest and part of the left arm. This very close proximity of the converging nerve fibres confuses the brain, which interprets the heart pain as coming from the chest area and left arm (and sometimes the neck or jaw). Figure 1.1 illustrates common areas where referred pain may be experienced.

Figure 1.1 Referred pain regions

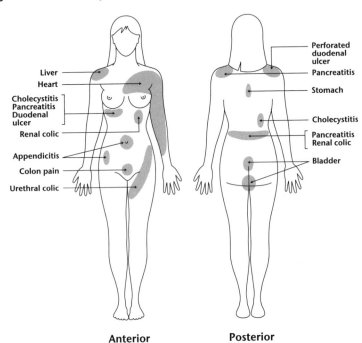

Anterior   Posterior

19 **A solid tumour is usually classified according to the *tissue* from which it originates.**

The majority of solid tumours arise from epithelial tissue which is the main type of tissue that lines the internal and external surfaces of the body's organs (for example, the lungs, colon and breasts). Tumours arising from epithelial tissues are called carcinomas. Haematological cancers are classified according to the blood cells from which they originate.

20 **Cancer cells can *metastasize* away from their origin.**

The metastasis of cancer cells is the movement or spread of the cells to other areas of the body and may occur in three ways:

I.   The growing mass of cells penetrates a blood or lymphatic vessel, enters the circulating blood or lymph and travels through either system. The cells can then settle in any organ or region of the body. Some types of cancer have sites they tend to metastasize to.
II. Cancerous cells can be spread during surgery.
III. They can spread to neighbouring organs – this is common in the GI tract because of the close proximity of organs.

There are many pathophysiological changes associated with the development of metastases. Sometimes it is only through the detection of such metastatic signs and symptoms that a cancer is diagnosed. Some common clinical signs of metastases include pleural effusion of the lungs which may indicate a metastasis in the lungs which is a common metastatic site for breast cancers (or it may be indicative of a primary lung tumour); ascites in the peritoneum can indicate metastasis in the peritoneal cavity which is a common metastatic site for ovarian cancers.

2 Inflammation, infection and immunity

INTRODUCTION

The immune system has three lines of defence: (1) physical and chemical barriers to infective agents; (2) the inflammatory response; and (3) the immune system reaction. When pathogens invade the body, there are two types of possible immune response that can occur: specific and non-specific.

Infection occurs when the body's defence mechanisms are invaded by pathogens. Inflammation is a protective attempt by the body to remove the inflammatory stimulus and initiate the healing process in the tissue. Inflammation can be classified as either acute or chronic. Acute inflammation is the initial response of the body to harmful stimuli while chronic (prolonged) inflammation causes a change in the type of cells which are present at the inflammation site. In the absence of inflammation, wounds and infections would never heal, causing progressive destruction of the tissue.

Immunodeficiency occurs when the immune system is less functional than normal, resulting in recurring and life-threatening infections. In contrast, autoimmune diseases are caused by a hyperactive immune system that attacks normal tissues as if they were foreign organisms. Hypersensitivity disorders are often caused by an overactive immune response.

Nurses need to recognize the characteristics of infection and inflammation to treat such conditions quickly and efficiently because certain infections can develop quickly and be life-threatening.

Useful resources

Nurses! Test Yourself in Anatomy and Physiology

Chapter 11

Ross and Wilson's Anatomy and Physiology in Health and Illness (11th edition)

Chapter 15

TRUE OR FALSE?

Are the following statements true or false?

1 For infection control, nurses should always wear gloves during patient contact.

2 Bacteria contain carbohydrates that may cause infection.

3 Fungi can be classified as yeasts or moulds.

4 Parasitic infections are very common in cold climates.

5 B-cells are responsible for humoral immunity.

6 Disorders of the immune system fall into three main categories.

MULTIPLE CHOICE

Identify one correct answer for each of the following.

7 Tonsillitis is most commonly caused by:

a) viruses

b) bacteria

c) fungi

d) protozoa

8 Pathogens can be transmitted via which of the following routes?

a) airborne

b) arthropods

c) direct and indirect contact

d) all of the above

9 Which of the following is a major protein system that supports the inflammatory response?

a) inflammation system

b) complimentary system

c) complement system

d) compliment system

FILL IN THE BLANKS

Fill in the blanks in each statement using the options in this box.
Not all of them are required, so choose carefully!

opportunistic	carcinogenesis
infection	T-
latent	B-
viral	

10 _____ can occur when a pathogen or disease-causing substance enters the body.

11 _____ infections occur when normal immune and inflammatory responses fail.

12 _____ infections usually occur in people with weakened immune systems.

13 In the cell-mediated immune response, _____cells respond directly to the foreign antigen.

MATCH THE TERMS

Classify each immune disorder listed below:

A. autoimmune

B. hypersensitivity

C. immunodeficiency

14 Anaphylaxis _____

15 HIV disease _____

16 Rheumatoid arthritis _____

17 Lupus erythematosus _____

18 Allergic rhinitis _____

ANSWERS

TRUE OR FALSE?

1 **For infection control, nurses should always wear gloves during patient contact.**

It is not always necessary to wear gloves during patient contact, sometimes they can actually be a mode of transmission for infection. The most effective infection control measure is a good hand-washing technique.

2 **Bacteria contain carbohydrates that may cause infection.**

Pathogenic bacteria contain two different types of proteins that cause infection: (1) exotoxins – released during growth; and (2) endotoxins – released when the bacterial cell wall breaks down. Endotoxins cause fevers and do not respond to antibiotics.

3 **Fungi can be classified as yeasts or moulds.**

Fungi are relatively large compared to other microorganisms. Yeasts are round, single cell organisms that can survive with or without oxygen. Moulds are filament-like organisms that require oxygen.

As part of its natural flora, the body has a range of fungi. However, sometimes they can overproduce, especially when the normal flora is unbalanced. Yeast infections sometimes occur during certain antibiotic treatments because the antibiotic will also attack the normal flora in addition to its bacterial target.

Most fungal infections (such as athlete's foot) are relatively minor unless the immune system is already compromised (for example, during cancer treatment) or if the infection spreads systemically.

4 **Parasitic infections are very common in cold climates.**

Infections caused by parasites are less common in cold climates but can be very prevalent in hot, moist climates. Most parasitic infections (such as tapeworms) occur in the GI tract. Parasites depend on their host for food and a protective environment, often to the detriment of the host's well-being.

5 **B-cells are responsible for humoral immunity.**

B-cells trigger the humoral (antibody)-mediated immune response. B-cells originate in the bone marrow and mature to become plasma cells that produce antibodies. Antibodies provide immunity by destroying bacteria and viruses before they enter host cells.

6 | **Disorders of the immune system fall into three main categories.**

The three types of immune disorders are:

I.   *autoimmune disorders* – when the body initiates an immune response on itself (as in rheumatoid arthritis).
II. *hypersensitivity disorders* – when an allergen enters the body and causes an over-sensitive immune reaction which may be instant or delayed.
III. *immunodeficiency disorders* – resulting from a suppressed or deficient immune system (such as AIDS, chronic fatigue syndrome (ME) or during cancer treatment).

 MULTIPLE CHOICE

Correct answers identified in bold italics

7 | **Tonsillitis is most commonly caused by:**

a) viruses   b) bacteria   c) fungi   d) protozoa

Tonsillitis is an infection most commonly caused by a virus, often those that frequently affect the respiratory system (such as the influenza virus), but it can also be caused by bacteria. Irrespective of the cause, the main symptom is a sore throat, often accompanied by red, swollen tonsils which may have visible pus-filled spots. As a result, the patient may have difficulty swallowing. The patient may also present with a headache, coughing, fatigue, pain in the ears and neck. If the tonsillitis is caused by a virus, there may be associated flu-like symptoms. If it is bacterial, the face may be flushed or have a rash. Most GPs will diagnose tonsillitis based on the symptoms, however, a throat swab may be taken if bacterial infection is suspected and in patients who are immune-compromised or where the infection is recurrent. For an isolated episode, the infection usually subsides within a few days and painkillers may be prescribed to ease symptoms. If the infection is known to be bacterial, an antibiotic may be prescribed to treat the infection. For recurrent infections, surgical removal of the tonsils (tonsillectomy) may be recommended.

8 | **Pathogens can be transmitted via which of the following routes?**

a) airborne   b) arthropods   c) direct and indirect contact
d) all of the above

When the body's first-line defence mechanisms are overcome by a pathogen, infection can occur. Pathogens can enter the body through the GI tract, the respiratory tract or through the skin. Transmission may be airborne or through direct or indirect contact, or pathogens may be spread by arthropods (such as flies, lice, mites).

9 **Which of the following is a major protein system that supports the inflammatory response?**

a) inflammation system   b) complimentary system
c) complement system   d) compliment system

The proteins of the complement system continuously circulate in the blood but are usually inactive. When an antigen of a pathogen is encountered by an antibody in the body, the proteins of the complement cascade become activated to initiate and support the inflammatory response. The complement cascade enhances the inflammatory response in two ways: (1) increasing vascular permeability; and (2) promoting chemotaxis (movement of white blood cells to the area of inflammation). It also supports the immune response by encouraging phagocytosis of the foreign bodies and helping breakdown of the foreign cell (cytolysis). *(Hint: to distinguish the spelling, think compl*e*ment (with an E)* e*nhances the inflammatory response.)*

FILL IN THE BLANKS

10 *Infection* **can occur when a pathogen or disease-causing substance enters the body.**

Infection results when the tissue-destroying microorganisms enter the body and multiply. Infections can result in a minor illness (for example, the common cold) but sometimes can induce more life-threatening conditions, such as septicaemia (blood poisoning). Septicaemia causes vasodilation and multiple organ dysfunction throughout the body.

11 *Viral* **infections can occur when normal immune and inflammatory responses fail.**

Viruses are intracellular parasites that contain genetic material but need a specific host cell to replicate inside. The virus replicates in the host cell using the host cell's DNA. It remains there undetected by the immune system until it is released and infects other cells.

12 *Opportunistic* **infections usually occur in people with weakened immune systems.**

When the immune system is weakened or compromised, this presents an 'opportunity' for pathogens to infect the body. Situations when the immune system may be weakened include therapeutic immunosuppression (following organ transplant), cancer treatment, antibiotic treatment as a result of malnutrition, AIDS patients and pregnancy.

13 **In the cell-mediated immune response, _T_-cells respond directly to the foreign antigen.**

T-cells respond directly to antigens on the cell surface of invading pathogens. Their response triggers the secretion of lymph proteins (called lymphokines) which destroy target cells such as virus-infected or cancer cells. T-cells can be classified as helper, killer or suppressor cells. Helper T-cells stimulate B-cells to mature into plasma cells which synthesize and secrete antibodies. Killer (or cytotoxic) T-cells bind to the cell surface of the invading pathogen and destroy them. Suppressor T-cells reduce the humoral-mediated immune response.

 MATCH THE TERMS

14 Anaphylaxis **B.** hypersensitivity

Anaphylaxis is an acute allergic reaction triggered by exposure to an antigen. Symptoms include sudden onset and rapid progression of urticaria (hives) and respiratory distress. A severe reaction can also cause vascular collapse, systemic shock and even death.

- *Causes:* There are many possible triggering antigens including vaccine serums, hormones, certain enzymes, anaesthetics, latex, foods, blood/blood products or sensitizing drugs – the most common being penicillin.

- *Pathophysiology:* Upon first exposure to the allergen, the immune system becomes sensitized to the allergen and produces specific antibodies (called immunoglobulin E, IgE) which remain on the surface of mast cells. In a second exposure to the allergen, the IgE molecules bind to the allergen and sensitize mast cells which degranulate and release histamine (and other inflammatory mediators). Histamine causes constriction of some smooth muscle, resulting in vasodilation and increased vascular permeability (Figure 2.1). In an anaphylactic reaction vasodilation is very rapid which causes a sudden drop in blood pressure; this is accompanied by contraction of smooth muscle in the respiratory airways which may result in wheezing and dyspnoea.

- *Signs and symptoms:* Immediately after exposure, patients may report a feeling of severe anxiety. This is accompanied by dyspnoea (shortness of breath), weakness, sweating and urticaria.

- *Diagnosis and treatment:* Take patient's history; note signs and symptoms; monitor heart rate, respiratory rate and blood pressure. An injection of adrenaline (epinephrine) should be administered, massage the site of injection to improve the drug distribution in the circulation; if the patient is unconscious, it can be administered by IV injection.

Figure 2.1 The mechanism of anaphylaxis

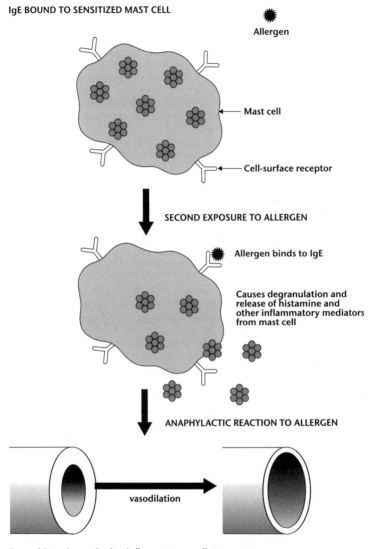

Excess histamine and other inflammatory mediators cause:

• smooth muscle constriction, resulting in bronchoconstriction;

• vasodilation which triggers sudden decrease in blood pressure;

• increased vascular permeability causing oedema and the appearance of hives.

15 HIV disease **C. immunodeficiency**

Infection with human immuno-deficiency virus (HIV) causes a progressive destruction of the acquired immune system, specifically the T-cells (T4 lymphocytes), meaning the immune response becomes impaired. The infection is characterized by repeated opportunistic infections that progressively weaken the immune system by destroying helper T-cells, therefore suppressing the acquired immune system. When the number of circulating helper T-cells becomes very low, opportunistic infections present a significant threat of serious disease. The patient is now said to have developed acquired immuno-deficiency syndrome (AIDS).

■ *Causes and risk factors:* HIV is transmitted in body fluids. Contact with infected blood, tissue, semen or vaginal fluids can cause infection. HIV can cross the placenta and infect a foetus; the newborn is also at risk of infection during delivery and via breast milk. It is thought that the levels of HIV in other body fluids such as saliva, urine, tears and faeces are insufficient to cause infection.

■ *Pathophysiology:* HIV requires a host cell to replicate. It destroys helper T-cells, causing a gradual reduction in the number of helper T-cells in the body, therefore weakening the body's acquired immune responses (cell-mediated and humoral). The average time between initial HIV infection and development of AIDS is 8–10 years.

■ *Signs and symptoms:* After initial exposure, an infected person may exhibit mild, flu-like symptoms or no symptoms at all. After this primary infection, an individual may remain asymptomatic (exhibit no symptoms) for up to 10 years. As the disease progresses, an infected individual may begin to exhibit opportunistic infections. Repeated opportunistic infections will overwhelm the weakened immune system and the patient develops AIDS. In children, the asymptomatic period is usually much shorter (averaging 17 months); the symptoms children exhibit are similar to those of adults.

■ *Diagnosis and treatment:* A person may remain negative for HIV antibodies for as long as 14 months after initial infection although a positive test for HIV antibodies is usually obtained 3–7 weeks post-exposure. Antibody tests in neonates can be unreliable due to the presence of maternal antibodies in the child for up to 18 months after birth – this can lead to false-positive results in neonatal tests. Routine blood tests monitor helper T-cell count and HIV viral load in the blood, these are used to evaluate the level of immunosuppression. There is no cure for HIV or AIDS but several drugs exist to slow the progression of the disease. Certain antiretroviral drugs (called highly active antiretroviral therapy, HAART treatment) reduce replication of the virus and hence slow HIV progression. Anti-infective drugs can also be prescribed to limit the number of opportunistic infections that will progressively weaken the immune system. Antineoplastic agents can be used to treat the rare cancers often associated with HIV and AIDS.

16 Rheumatoid arthritis   **A. autoimmune**

A chronic, systemic, inflammatory autoimmune disorder causing destruction of the peripheral joints and surrounding muscles, tendons, ligaments and blood vessels. Rheumatoid arthritis (RA) patients can undergo spontaneous remission but also unpredictable exacerbation of their condition. It is more prevalent in females than males and usually affects patients between the ages of 20 and 50.

- *Causes and risk factors:* The cause remains unknown but genetic influences, hormones and infections are thought to be involved. Viruses are thought to trigger RA in people who have a genetic susceptibility for the disease.

- *Pathophysiology:* Exposure to an antigen triggers the formation of altered antibodies that the body does not recognize as its own. Since they are recognized as foreign, the body then forms another antibody against them, called rheumatoid factor, which causes inflammation. This inflammation eventually causes cartilage damage. The continued immune response includes activation of the complement cascade which stimulates release of inflammatory mediators and this exacerbates joint destruction.

- *Signs and symptoms:* Initially symptoms are non-specific, including fatigue, malaise, weight loss and persistent low-grade fever. As the inflammation progresses more specific symptoms are observed such as swelling around the joint which may be warm and/or painful. These symptoms occur particularly in the fingers, but also in wrists, elbows, knees and ankles.

- *Diagnosis and treatment:* No test will provide a definitive diagnosis of RA but there are useful indicative tests:
  - X-ray – soft-tissue swelling and bone demineralization are observable and X-rays can be used to determine extent of cartilage and bone destruction.
  - Testing for presence of rheumatoid factor – although this is not sufficient to diagnose the disease, it is useful in determining prognosis. The prognosis worsens as nodules and vasculitis (inflammation of blood or lymph vessels) develops.

Since it is a chronic illness RA usually requires lifelong treatment and sometimes surgery on joints that are painful or damaged. Treatments to reduce pain and inflammation help to maintain quality of life. Non-steroidal anti-inflammatory drugs (NSAIDs) are the main type of painkiller used since they decrease inflammation and relieve joint pain. Immunosuppressants are sometimes used early in the disease to halt its progression. Tumour necrosis factor (TNF) alpha-blockers are a relatively new class of drug that is proving effective in treating adults and children with RA and other autoimmune disorders. Patients are also encouraged to practise certain exercises to maintain joint function.

17 Lupus erythematosus   **A. autoimmune**

A chronic, inflammatory, autoimmune disorder affecting the connective tissues. There are two forms of lupus erythematosus: systemic and discoid. Systemic lupus erythematosus (SLE) affects multiple organs and can be fatal, it is the more common form of the condition. It is more common in females, particular those of Afro-Caribbean origin. Discoid lupus erythematosus only affects the skin.

- *Causes:* The exact cause of SLE is unknown. It is thought to be a combination of genetic and environmental factors. Possible triggers include viruses, infection, stress, prolonged use of medication, sunlight exposure, hormones and endocrine changes (including puberty, menopause and childbirth).

- *Pathophysiology:* The body produces antibodies against its own cells which suppress its normal immune responses. A feature of SLE is that patients produce antibodies against many different types of its own tissues such as red blood cells, white blood cells, platelets and even its own organs.

- *Signs and symptoms:* Symptoms of lupus can vary. Some people only experience a mild form of the condition, whereas others are more severely affected and may develop serious complications. As with other autoimmune disorders, there are no specific symptoms. SLE primarily causes fatigue, joint pain and skin rashes (particularly the 'butterfly rash' over the cheeks and bridge of the nose), as the immune system attacks the body's tissue and cells. Certain blood disorders may be detected such as anaemia, leucopenia, lymphopenia and thrombocytopenia. An elevated erythrocyte sedimentation rate (ESR) may also occur.

- *Diagnosis and treatment:* SLE can be difficult to diagnose because symptoms vary between patients. Active disease is diagnosed by decreased serum complement levels since complement levels decrease during active SLE episodes.

Drugs are the main form of treatment for SLE. In mild conditions, NSAIDs are sufficient to control the arthritis and joint pain. Topical corticosteroids can be applied to treat skin lesions. Hydroxychloroquine (normally used to treat malaria) is also effective in treating some symptoms of SLE, such as skin rashes, joint and muscle pain and fatigue, although there can be complications associated with this type of medication. Patients are also advised to protect themselves from the sun.

18 Allergic rhinitis   **B. hypersensitivity**

When airborne allergens are inhaled, they may trigger an immune response in the upper airway, which may cause inflammation of the nasal mucous membranes (rhinitis) or conjunctivitis (inflammation of the membrane lining inside the eyelids and covering the eyeball). Seasonal allergic rhinitis is commonly known as hay fever.

- *Causes:* The airborne allergens that trigger the disorder include dust, animal fibres, pollen (triggers hay fever) or work-related allergens (such as flour, chemical vapours or latex).

- *Pathophysiology:* Allergic rhinitis is a hypersensitivity response to an environmental allergen. The nasal and mucous membranes swell and may lead to secondary sinus or middle ear infections. Complications include pneumonia or bronchitis.

- *Signs and symptoms:* This can cause cold-like symptoms, such as sneezing and runny nose; patients may also experience headache or sinus pain and have an itchy throat. Dark circles may develop under the eyes as a result of venous congestion in the maxillary sinuses.

- *Diagnosis and treatment:* Analysis of nasal secretions may show elevated levels of the white blood cells. The best advice for any allergy involves controlling symptoms and avoiding allergens known to trigger infection. Antihistamines are the main type of drug prescribed to reduce the runny nose and watery eyes symptoms. However, some antihistamines can have undesired sedative effects, although non-sedating antihistamines are also available.

3 The integumentary system

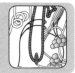

INTRODUCTION

The skin is a complex organ consisting of three distinct layers (epidermis, dermis and subcutaneous) and accessory structures, such as hair and nails. When intact, the skin provides the body's first line of defence as well as controlling body temperature and preventing excessive fluid loss.

Due to the prominence of the skin, its integrity is under constant threat. Skin disorders can be due to many factors such as trauma, allergy, infection, tumour, or environmental stresses. They may also be degenerative, congenital or secondary to another illness or disease within another organ system. For example, acne can be attributed to a hormonal imbalance in the endocrine system but appears as lesions on the skin. Diagnosis of skin disorders sometimes involves taking a sample of affected tissue or collecting fluid from a lesion. Sensitivity patch testing on the skin is commonly used in allergy investigations.

Increasingly, the skin is used as an administrative route for drugs such as topical gels to relieve pain or inflammation; or transdermal administration in nicotine replacement therapy or treatment of motion sickness.

The visibility of the skin, hair and nails makes them useful when assessing many conditions, with the characteristics of skin lesions being helpful when making a diagnosis. Furthermore, many nursing interventions involve the skin so nurses should know and understand how the skin protects the body, helps maintain homoeostasis.

Useful resources

Nurses! Test Yourself in Anatomy and Physiology

Chapter 3

Symptoms, Diagnosis and Treatment

Chapter 7

American Academy of Dermatology

http://www.aad.org

LABELLING EXERCISE

1–5 Identify the type of skin lesions in Figure 3.1, using the terms in the box below:

vesicle	papule
ulcer	weal
pustule	

Figure 3.1 Skin lesions

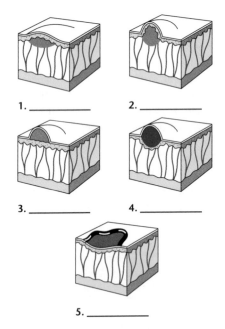

1. _____   2. _____

3. _____   4. _____

5. _____

TRUE OR FALSE?

Are the following statements true or false?

6 Impetigo is an autoimmune condition.

7 Laser therapy can be used in the treatment of warts.

8 A partial-thickness burn affects only the epidermis.

9 Severe neuralgia is a frequent complication of the herpes simplex infection.

10 Papular urticaria may be life-threatening.

11 There are three basic types of skin cancer.

12 Infection by the *Varicella zoster* virus leads to chickenpox.

13 A burrow is the primary lesion of *Varicella zoster*.

14 Scabies is caused by a parasitic infection.

15 In a closed wound, the epithelium remains intact.

MULTIPLE CHOICE

Identify one correct answer for each of the following.

16 What abnormal skin colour might indicate rising levels of bilirubin?

a) yellow

b) blue

c) red

d) general paleness

17 Androgenetic alopecia can be treated with:

a) oestrogens

b) benzyl penicillin

c) topical minoxidil

d) spirolactone

18 An emollient is:

a) an antibiotic

b) a steroid

c) an alcohol-based medication

d) a substance that moisturizes and soothes skin.

19 The stages of deep wound healing occur in which order?

a) migration, inflammation, proliferation and maturation

b) inflammation, proliferation, migration and maturation

c) inflammation, proliferation, maturation and migration

d) inflammation, migration, proliferation and maturation

20 Moles may be considered sinister if:

a) they increase in size

b) they change in shape

c) they bleed

d) any of the above occur

21 Which of these are not risk factors for malignant melanoma?

a) exposure to sunlight

b) dark skin

c) history of sunburn

d) family history

22 Which application is best for treating acute oozing skin conditions?

a) drying lotions

b) powders

c) ointments

d) creams

23 Onychomycosis refers to:

a) ringworm of the scalp

b) inflammation of sebaceous glands

c) a fungal infection of the nail bed

d) an area of necrotic tissue

24 Treatment of chronic urticaria includes the application of:

a) corticosteroids

b) antihistamines

c) menthol cream

d) all of the above

25 Which of the following is not part of the primary treatment for full-thickness burns?

    a) maintaining cosmetic appearance of skin

    b) replacing lost fluids and electrolytes

    c) providing dietary nutrients

    d) preventing infection

26 An open wound is an injury that causes a break in which skin layer?

    a) all skin layers

    b) epidermis

    c) dermis

    d) subcutaneous

MATCH THE TERMS

Match each skin disorder with a possible cause from the following list:

A. bacterial infection   **C.** fungal infection

B. viral infection   **D.** inflammation

27	Cellulitis	_____
28	Oral thrush	_____
29	Psoriasis	_____
30	Shingles	_____
31	Athlete's foot	_____
32	Impetigo	_____
33	Eczema	_____

ANSWERS

LABELLING EXERCISE

Figure 3.2 Skin lesions

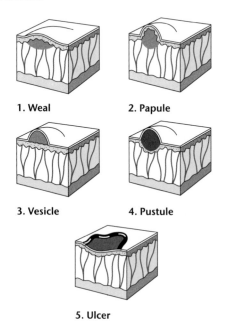

1. Weal

2. Papule

3. Vesicle

4. Pustule

5. Ulcer

1 *Weal (wheal):* a localized elevation of the epidermis caused by an accumulation of fluid in the papillary dermis. An example of a weal lesion is urticaria (hives).

2 *Papule:* a solid elevation of both the dermis and epidermal layers that contains fluid. An insect bite may cause a papule to develop. Nodules are large papules that sometimes extend into the subcutaneous layer, for example, a cyst.

3 *Vesicle (blister):* a papule located directly under the skin surface that has filled with fluid. A large vesicle is sometimes called a bulla (pl. bullae). Partial thickness (second degree) burns often form vesicles.

4 | **Pustule:** a lesion similar in size to a papule but filled with pus which contains necrotic inflammatory cells. An acne blemish is an example of a pustule.

5 | **Ulcer (erosion):** can occur after a vesicle or pustule ruptures. Ulcers have lost at least part of the epidermis. Examples include pressure (bed) sores (also known as decubitis ulcers).

TRUE OR FALSE?

6 | **Impetigo is an autoimmune condition.**

Impetigo is a highly contagious bacterial skin infection of the superficial layers of the skin that is most common in children (about 70 per cent of cases occur in children, making it the most common childhood skin infection in the UK). It is caused by the *Staphylococcus aureus* or more rarely *Streptococcus pyogenes* bacteria. The first sign of impetigo is a patch of red, itchy skin.

The condition is characterized by red sores, generally around the mouth and nose. The sores soon burst and ooze fluid or pus, forming a yellowish-brown crust, which leaves a red mark as it dries. The condition usually heals without scarring. Although the sores are not painful, they may be very itchy. To prevent the spread of infection (to other body parts or other people), it is important not to touch or scratch the affected area. Treatment is usually with topical or oral antibiotics and good hygiene. In rare cases, symptoms may be more severe and the patient may develop a fever and swollen glands.

7 | **Laser therapy can be used in the treatment of warts.**

Warts are benign lesions of the skin caused by the human papillomavirus (HPV), which most commonly occurs in children and young adults. The infection is acquired when the virus is introduced into the skin through defects in the epidermis. New treatments for warts involve using a pulsed dye laser which selectively destroys warts without damaging the surrounding skin. The laser selectively destroys blood vessels that supply the wart, as well as thermally destroying the wart. Traditional treatments for warts involve physical destruction of the virally infected cell. These treatments include the application of acids (such as salicylic acid), liquid nitrogen therapy (cryosurgery), electrocautery and carbon dioxide ablation. Such treatments all cause destruction of the top layer of the skin and may result in permanent scarring. In many cases, warts may be resistant to these kinds of therapy. Compared with alternative treatments, pulsed dye laser therapy is very safe and effective, even in warts that have become resistant to previous treatment.

8 | **A partial-thickness burn affects only the epidermis.**

In recent years, classification of burns by burn depth has changed. Injury to the epidermis (top or outer skin layer) is now called a superficial burn (formerly called a first degree burn). Injury to the dermis (second layer) is now called a partial-thickness or dermal injury (formerly second degree). An injury that extends down to the third layer (the subcutaneous tissue, which includes fat) is called a full-thickness injury (formerly third degree). Burns that damage muscles underneath the subcutaneous skin layer are described as full-thickness burns (formerly fourth degree). Full-thickness burns tend to be less painful than superficial and partial-thickness burns because the sensory nerves may have been damaged or destroyed by a full-thickness burn.

Superficial burns normally heal within 5–7 days. A common type of superficial burn is sunburn. Since the epidermis is thin (about the thickness of a piece of paper), it is easily replaced. Even when skin is not injured, the epidermis is completely replaced every 45 to 75 days. Healing from a superficial burn usually occurs without scarring, although there may be some permanent discolouration. The dermis is 15–40 times thicker than the epidermis, therefore the seriousness of a partial thickness (or dermal) burn depends on the depth to which the dermis has been injured. Partial-thickness burns usually leave scars. Deep and large partial-thickness burns will usually require skin grafting. A full-thickness burn destroys all three layers of skin, resulting in the loss of not only the skin but also the accessory structures such as hair follicles, sweat glands, and the region where new skin cells are formed. For these reasons, full-thickness burns require skin grafts. Fourth degree burns extend through the skin into underlying tissues, such as ligaments and muscle; these are often life-threatening.

9 | **Severe neuralgia is a frequent complication of the herpes simplex infection.**

Although neuralgia can occur after infection with the herpes simplex virus (HSV), it is generally mild and gives little cause for concern. However, other neurological syndromes have been linked to HSV infection, including epilepsy, multiple sclerosis, atypical pain syndromes, and ascending or transverse myelitis (inflammation of the spinal column). These are typically more serious.

10 | **Papular urticaria may be life-threatening.**

Urticaria is the clinical name for hives. Papules may open when scratched and become crusty and infected. Papular urticaria is a common disorder in children, manifested by chronic or recurrent papules caused by an allergic hypersensitivity reaction to insects (for example, mosquitoes). Treatment is usually with oral antihistamines and oral corticosteroids, such as prednisolone.

11 **There are three basic types of skin cancer.**

Skin cancers account for about 40 per cent of all cancers. In recent years there has been a significant increase in the number of reported cases. Basal cell carcinoma and squamous cell carcinoma are the two most common types of skin cancer. The third type, malignant melanoma, is a less frequent but more serious form of skin cancer representing 4 per cent of all skin cancer cases but around 80 per cent of all skin cancer deaths.

Exposure to ultraviolet (UV) radiation causes most skin cancers by triggering genetic mutations. Areas of skin with wide exposure to the sun are at significant risk of skin cancer but protection from the sun significantly reduces risk. As with other cancers, skin cancer lesions progress through the stages of initiation, and promotion, progression and metastasis.

12 **Infection by the *Varicella zoster* virus leads to chickenpox.**

Chickenpox is a highly contagious illness caused by primary infection with the *Varicella zoster* virus. It usually starts with a vesicle skin rash, mainly on the body and head rather than at the periphery, and this develops into itchy raw lesions which mostly heal without scarring. Chickenpox is rarely fatal, although it is generally more severe in adult males than in adult females or children. Pregnant women and those with a suppressed immune system are at highest risk of serious complications. Chickenpox is now believed to be the cause of one-third of stroke cases in children. The most common future complication of chickenpox is shingles, caused by reactivation of the *Varicella zoster* virus decades after the initial episode of chickenpox. Following primary infection, there is usually lifelong protective immunity from further episodes of chickenpox.

13 **A burrow is the primary lesion of *Varicella zoster*.**

The primary lesions associated with *Varicella zoster* infection are small blister-like vesicles that are a characteristic of chickenpox. A person with chickenpox is infectious from 1–5 days before the rash appears. The contagious period continues until all the blisters have formed scabs, which may take 5–10 days. It takes from 10–21 days after contact with an infected person for someone to develop chickenpox. In adults, chickenpox is often associated with loss of appetite (anorexia), myalgia, nausea, fever, headache, sore throat, earache, feeling pressure in the head or swollen face and malaise. In children, the first symptom is usually the appearance of a papular rash, followed by development of malaise, fever and loss of appetite. Less common symptoms include cough, rhinitis, abdominal pain and gastrointestinal distress. Typically, the disease is more severe in adults. Burrows are a sign of infestation by scabies-causing parasites.

14 **Scabies is caused by a parasitic infection.**

Scabies is a contagious skin infection caused by tiny parasitic mites that burrow into the skin and lay eggs. Symptoms include intense itch (sometimes worse at night) and skin rash indicating where the mites have burrowed. Diagnosis is usually from observing the skin although a skin sample may be taken and examined for the parasitic mites and their eggs. Insecticide creams are the used to treat the parasitic infection, with permethrin cream usually recommended as the first treatment option, however, it should only be used under medical supervision if pregnant or breast-feeding and in children under 2 years. Malathion lotion is used if the permethrin cream is ineffective, it has no known effects during pregnancy and breast-feeding. Treating scabies also involves educating patients properly about correct hygiene to limit the spread of infection. Scabies tends to be more common where lots of people are living in close proximity, such as schools and nursing homes.

15 **In a closed wound, the epithelium remains intact.**

Closed wounds can affect any internal tissue but the epithelium is intact and so infection is less likely to occur. A common example of a closed wound is a bruise (contusion) which is caused by bleeding in the dermis. A facial contusion may be relatively harmless or can indicate more serious internal injury such as intracranial bleeding. Closed wounds affecting organs or organ systems are often life-threatening.

MULTIPLE CHOICE

Correct answers identified in bold italics

16 **What abnormal skin colour might indicate rising levels of bilirubin?**

a) yellow   b) blue   c) red   d) general paleness

A yellow colouring in skin indicates the presence of jaundice as a result of increased bilirubin levels in blood. Except for physiological jaundice in the newborn, this condition does not normally occur. The condition in the child or adult may be first noted in the junction of the hard and soft palate in the mouth and in the sclera (whites) of the eyes. As levels of serum bilirubin rise, jaundice becomes more evident over the rest of the body.

Other skin colours indicate a range of abnormal physiological states:

- Erythema, an intense redness of the skin, is often associated with inflammation or fever and is related to an increased rate of blood flow through the surface vessels.

- Cyanosis is characterized by a bluish colour and often signifies decreased tissue perfusion that may be due to anaemia or inadequate blood flow.

- General paleness (pallor) may indicate acute anxiety or fear, and results from the peripheral vasoconstriction that occurs with sympathetic nervous system stimulation. Skin can also appear pale due to vasoconstriction from exposure to cold or pallor may be caused by oedema.

17 **Androgenetic alopecia can be treated with:**

a) oestrogens   b) benzyl penicillin   *c) topical minoxidil*
d) spirolactone

Androgenetic (or androgenic) alopecia is a degenerative skin disorder affecting males and females. Minoxidil is a vasodilator medication that slows or stops hair loss and promotes hair regrowth. It is available over the counter for treatment of androgenetic alopecia, among other hair loss treatments, but measurable changes disappear within months after discontinuation of treatment.

The mechanism by which minoxidil promotes hair growth is not fully understood. Minoxidil is also a vasodilator. It is speculated that by widening blood vessels and opening potassium channels, it allows more blood, and therefore oxygen and nutrients, to enter the follicle. It is less effective when there is a large area of hair loss. In addition, its effectiveness has largely been demonstrated in younger men (18–41 years). Minoxidil use is indicated for central (vertex) hair loss only.

18 **An emollient is:**

a) an antibiotic   b) a steroid   c) an alcohol-based medication
d) a substance that moisturizes and soothes skin

An emollient is an agent that soothes and softens the skin such as lanolin or liquid paraffin. Emollients are used alone as moisturizers to reduce the need for active drug therapy (such as corticosteroids for eczema) and in skin preparations as a base for more active drugs, such as antibiotics.

19 **The stages in deep wound healing occur in which order?**

a) migration, inflammation, proliferation and maturation
b) inflammation, proliferation, migration and maturation
c) inflammation, proliferation, maturation and migration
d) inflammation, migration, proliferation and maturation

Deep wound healing involves a number of phases and is more complex than primary or epidermal healing which is repaired by enlargement and migration of basal cells, contact inhibition and division of migrating and stationary basal cells.

In deep wound healing, the initial phase involves inflammation, a vascular and cellular response that prepares tissue for repair. During the inflammatory phase, a blood clot forms in the wound, uniting the damaged tissue edges. Vasodilation and increased permeability of blood vessels enhance the delivery of white cells that remove microbes and debris and mesenchymal cells which develop into fibroblasts.

In the subsequent migration phase, the clot develops into a scab and epithelial cells migrate beneath the scab to bridge the wound. Newly formed fibroblasts migrate along fibrin threads and begin producing scar tissue containing collagen and glycoproteins. Damaged blood vessels also begin to grow at this stage.

The proliferation phase is characterized by an extensive growth of epithelial cells beneath the scab, further deposition of collagen fibres and continued blood vessel growth.

The final maturation phase involves the sloughing off of the scab once the epidermis is restored to normal thickness. Collagen fibres become more organized in their pattern of deposition and fibroblasts decrease in number.

Scar tissue formation is called fibrosis. Depending on the extent of the wound, excess scar tissue may be formed resulting in raised scar formation which may remain within the boundaries of the original wound (hypertrophic scar) or it may extend into surrounding normal tissues (keloid scar). Scar tissue differs from normal skin since it frequently has fewer blood vessels and contains no hair, glandular tissue or sensory neurones.

20 **Moles are considered sinister if:**

a) they increase in size   b) they change in shape   c) they bleed
d) any of the above occur

Moles (or nevi) are defined as proliferation of melanocytes. Normally they are brownish in colour, flat or slightly raised, have smooth borders and have a uniform pigmentation. They are normally less than 6 mm in diameter. Abnormal characteristics of moles include asymmetry, changes in the border and colour, increased diameter and elevation, or bleeding from the mole. If any of these changes develop, patients should seek medical advice since it may indicate a malignant melanoma.

Malignant melanomas are the most prevalent life-threatening cancer in middle-aged adults. These cancers metastasize rapidly and have an extremely poor prognosis. Early recognition of cutaneous melanomas can have a major positive impact on surgical cure.

21 **Which of these are not risk factors for malignant melanoma?**

a) exposure to sunlight   *b) dark skin*   c) history of sunburn
d) family history

Melanoma is a malignant tumour of the skin that is increasing in frequency. Risk factors for the disease include a genetic predisposition, exposure to UV light (from sun or artificial sunbeds), steroid hormone activity, a fair complexion that burns easily in the sun and freckles. Wearing a sun lotion with a high sun protection factor (SPF) will help reduce skin damage from UV light. Melanomas arise as a result of malignant degeneration of melanocytes located in the basal layer of the epidermis.

LIBRARY, UNIVERSITY OF CHESTER

22 **Which application is best for treating acute oozing skin conditions?**

a) drying lotions b) powders c) ointments d) creams

Drying lotions are usually applied to acute oozing or weeping skin lesions. The most commonly used lotions contain alcohol, propylene glycol, polyethylene glycol or water. These lotions are convenient to apply and tend to dry rather than moisturize the skin. However, depending on the vehicle used, these lotions can be irritating to the skin, particularly when those containing alcohol and propylene glycol are applied to open wounds. The opposite of drying lotions is emollients which are used to moisturize dry skin conditions such as dermatitis (eczema) or psoriasis.

23 **Onychomycosis refers to:**

a) ringworm of the scalp   b) inflammation of sebaceous glands
c) a fungal infection of the nail bed   d) an area of necrotic tissue

Onychomycosis (fungal nail infection) is the most common disease of the nails and contributes to about a half of all nail abnormalities. It may affect toenails or fingernails, but toenail infections are particularly common. Symptoms include a thickened, yellow, or cloudy nail-plate. The nails can become rough and crumbly, or can separate from the nail bed. There is usually no pain or other symptoms, unless the disease is severe but patients with onychomycosis may experience significant psychosocial problems due to the appearance of the nail, particularly when fingernails are affected.

The pathogen that commonly causes onychomycosis is the yeast *Candida*, which enters a damaged or cracked nail. It is more common in older people. Treating onychomycosis is challenging because the infection is embedded within the nail and is difficult to reach. As a result full eradication of symptoms is very slow and may take a year or more. Most treatments are either systemic antifungal medications such as terbinafine and itraconazole, or topical such as nail paints containing salicylic acid, tioconazole or amorolfine. There is also evidence for combining systemic and topical treatments. Newer therapies include treatment with laser light sources which kill the fungus in the nail bed.

24 **Treatment of chronic urticaria includes the application of:**

a) corticosteroids   b) antihistamines   c) menthol cream
d) all of the above

Urticaria is the clinical name for hives which appear as an area of raised erythema and oedema of the superficial dermis and are frequently associated with type I hypersensitivity reactions. The lesions are mediated by release of histamine and may appear as weals, welts or hives. Chronic urticaria can be treated with antihistamines, corticosteroids and menthol cream. Patients should also be advised to avoid triggers where possible.

25 **Which of the following is not part of the primary treatment for full-thickness burns?**

a) maintaining cosmetic appearance of skin   b) replacing lost fluids and electrolytes   c) providing dietary nutrients   d) preventing infection

Most full-thickness burns cause severe damage to the skin and so often require skin grafts at a later stage because the skin cannot replace itself. Lots of fluids are lost by burns patients, therefore replacing fluids and electrolytes is very important in their treatment. Fluids are also important for thermoregulation to maintain an optimum body temperature. Nutrition is very important to provide the correct nutrients and energy for healing and also for thermoregulation. Infection control is essential because the broken skin provides an opportunity for invading pathogens to enter the body. Widespread infection can cause septicaemia which is the main cause of death in burns patients.

26 **An open wound is an injury that causes a break in which skin layer?**

a) all skin layers   *b) epidermis*   c) dermis   d) subcutaneous

An open wound is exposed to the external environment, meaning the outer epidermal layer has been broken. In a closed wound (such as a bruise), the epidermis remains intact. A number of types of open wounds exist (Figure 3.3).

I.   *Abrasion:* superficial wound over a large area usually caused by scraping against a solid object. There may be only slight bleeding which leaves this type of wound open to infection.
II. *Avulsion:* considerable amount of tissue is torn away with great force. It is usually associated with amputation injuries where considerable bleeding and serious internal damage may occur.
III. *Incision:* linear cut by sharp object (such as a knife wound). Bleeding can be severe if deep vessels are severed but such bleeding can help clean the wound and limit infection. It is usually stitched or bandaged to close the incision and limit the opportunity for infection.
IV. *Laceration:* caused by impact from a solid object. Tissue damage is more extensive because of the irregular, jagged tear. Despite extensive bleeding, there is a high risk of infection. Tissue often scars because it is difficult to correctly reposition lacerated tissue for healing.
V.   *Puncture:* Caused by slender, pointed objects, a puncture produces minimal bleeding therefore any invading pathogens can easily enter the body and cause infection.

Figure 3.3 Common open wounds

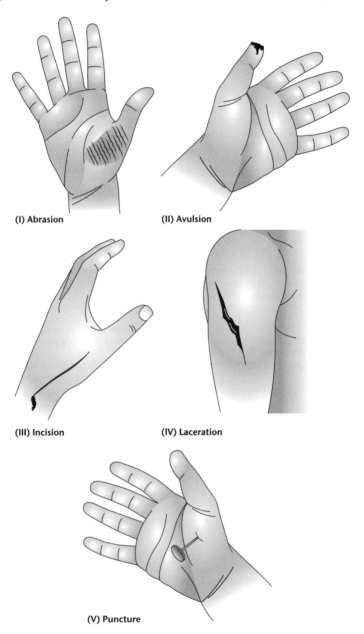

(I) Abrasion

(II) Avulsion

(III) Incision

(IV) Laceration

(V) Puncture

MATCH THE TERMS

27 Cellulitis   **A.** bacterial infection

- *Pathophysiology*: Cellulitis is an infection of the dermis and subcutaneous tissues usually caused by *Staphylococcus* or *Streptococci* bacteria.

- *Causes and risk factors*: A skin wound such as an ulcer, boil (furuncle) or carbuncle (abscess larger than a boil) can allow bacteria to enter the deeper tissues, causing infection and inflammation. Risk factors include diabetes mellitus, oedema and peripheral vascular disease.

- *Symptoms*: Hot, red, swollen and painful area, with itching, burning and tenderness as the infection develops. This may be accompanied by fever and chills as the bacteria release their toxins. There may be a clear line observed where the cellulitis stops but spreading of this can be observed as the infection spreads. Oozing and pus at the wound site can occur but this is less common.

- *Diagnosis and treatment*: Diagnosis is usually made by assessing the symptoms. If there is an open wound, a sample may be taken to identify the bacteria. Systemic antibiotics are required to treat the infection which can become severe and even life-threatening if left untreated.

- *Complications*: Certain individuals are more susceptible to cellulitis such as diabetics and immune-compromised patients. If the infection enters the blood, the patient is at risk of septicaemia (blood poisoning) which can be fatal if not treated urgently.

28 Oral thrush   **C.** fungal infection

- *Pathophysiology*: Oral thrush (candidiasis) is a fungal infection describing the presence of the *Candida* fungus in the mucous membranes of the mouth.

- *Risk factors*: It occurs more commonly in infants than adults although it is unusual for breast-fed infants to develop oral thrush. For bottle-fed babies, all teats should be replaced to reduce recurrence of infection. In adults and older children, it is less common although it can be common in denture-wearers. Mouth care is particularly important in chemotherapy patients and patients who receive radiotherapy to the head and neck. Certain antibiotics and other medications (such as steroids for asthma) can also be a risk factor.

- *Symptoms*: Formation of creamy white spots (plaques) in the mouth that when scraped off reveal shallow ulcers. The underlying mucous membrane is red and tender and may bleed when plaques are removed.

The tongue may also have a dense white coating. Babies may drool saliva or refuse to eat while adults may experience soreness or a burning sensation in the mouth.

- *Diagnosis and treatment*: Oral thrush is usually diagnosed by simply looking in the mouth. It generally responds quickly to antifungal treatments such as miconazole gel, drops or pastilles. In adults and older children predisposing causes should be investigated and treated first to prevent recurrence.

29 Psoriasis   **D. inflammation**

- *Pathophysiology*: Psoriasis is a chronic inflammatory skin disorder that is a form of hyperkeratosis which is characterized by excessive production of keratin when skin cells replace themselves too quickly. The life cycle to grow and replace normal skin cells is approximately 28 days. In psoriasis this cycle is accelerated, occurring as rapidly as every 2–6 days, meaning dead cells accumulate on the skin surface which produces the characteristic scaly patches. There are a number of different types of psoriasis but the most common is plaque psoriasis which accounts for the majority of cases.

- *Risk factors*: Plaque psoriasis is not contagious although there is a strong genetic link. Patients tend to become familiar with the triggers that cause their condition to flare up. Triggers include stress, smoking, alcohol, certain medicines (such as ibuprofen) and in response to skin injuries such as sunburn.

- *Causes*: These are not well known although there is evidence to suggest psoriasis is due to an autoimmune response that attacks healthy skin cells and speeds up the cycle of cell replication.

- *Symptoms*: Red, flaky crusty patches of skin covered in silver scales. Patches are usually quite small and can appear anywhere on the body although it is more common on the knees, elbows and scalp. Psoriasis can itch but it is not usually severe.

- *Diagnosis and treatment*: Diagnosis is usually by symptoms and determining if there is a family history. In rare cases, a skin sample may be taken to determine the type of psoriasis and to exclude other possible conditions. There is no cure for psoriasis so treatment is aimed at easing symptoms using topical emollient creams to moisturize skin. In more severe cases phototherapy using UV light can help reduce symptoms but this should be conducted under medical supervision.

30 Shingles   **B. viral infection**

- *Pathophysiology*: Shingles (herpes zoster) describes an infection of a nerve and its surrounding tissue. Shingles is characterized by a skin rash of tiny but painful fluid-filled blisters. It can affect any part of the body, including the face.

- *Risk factors*: Patients must previously have been infected with the *Varicella zoster* virus (usually during an episode of chickenpox).

The virus remains dormant in the body after the illness but can be reactivated later in life. Reactivation of the virus is thought to be associated with reduced immunity, therefore immuno-compromised patients are at risk. Stress is also a risk factor.

- *Causes*: It is caused by the *Varicella zoster* virus which also causes chickenpox although it is not triggered by exposure to the virus. After having chickenpox, the virus remains dormant in the body but can be reactivated later, causing shingles. Unlike chickenpox, shingles is not contagious. However, if someone who has never had chickenpox is in contact with shingles, they can catch the virus from the shingles patient and develop chickenpox.

- *Symptoms*: The initial symptoms include pain and paraesthesia (pins and needles), followed by red rash that develops on the face, neck, shoulders and back (similar to the chickenpox rash). Scabs form over the blisters that can scar if scratched. The rash usually takes 2–4 weeks to disappear. These symptoms can be accompanied by exhaustion. Local symptoms are alleviated with cool compresses or calamine lotion. Persistent pain may be a debilitating complication of this condition, particularly in the older adult.

- *Diagnosis and treatment*: Diagnosis is usually from symptoms, there is not usually any formal testing, however, if the condition affects the eyes, a patient may be referred. Treatment is aimed at easing symptoms. Rash and scabs should be kept clean and dry. Patients should wear loose clothing to reduce itching which can be treated topically with calamine lotion or orally with antihistamines. Paracetamol or ibuprofen can be used to treat mild–moderate pain, with opioids (such as codeine) being prescribed for more severe pain. Antiviral medications such as aciclovir help reduce the severity of the illness by stopping the virus from spreading, however they are most effective if taken within three days of the rash appearing.

- *Complications*: There is risk of the blisters becoming infected, particularly if scratched a lot. Other complications include encephalitis (inflammation of the brain), transverse myelitis (inflammation of the spinal cord) or severe persistent nerve pain (neuralgia).

31 Athlete's foot　　　　　　　　　　**C. fungal infection**

- *Pathophysiology*: Athlete's foot (tinea pedis) is a mild superficial fungal infection of foot and is quite common in adults. It causes a rash to develop, particularly between the toes but it can spread to the nail.

- *Causes*: It is caused by fungi that grow in warm, moist conditions.

- *Risk factors*: Athlete's foot is highly contagious and is associated with showers and swimming pools.

- *Symptoms*: An itchy, flaky rash between the toes which can smell. Deep cracks (fissures) can develop in the skin extending from the epidermis into the dermis, exposing new tissue which can be painful and increases the risk of bacterial infection. Symptoms usually disappear in 10 days when treated.

- *Diagnosis and treatment*: Mild infection is usually diagnosed by observing of the skin of the foot (sometimes with a UV light). Mild infections can be treated with over-the-counter antifungal (miconazole or clotrimazole) powders and creams. For more severe symptoms, a sample may be taken and treatment may include both topical and systemic antifungal medication. A severe rash may also need a hydrocortisone cream.

- *Complications*: Infection can spread to the toenail which can become infected with bacteria. This can lead to cellulitis.

32 Impetigo **A. bacterial infection**

- *Pathophysiology*: Impetigo is a superficial lesion of the skin caused by *Staphylococcus* or *Streptococci* bacteria. There are two types of impetigo: non-bullous or bullous lesions. Non-bullous accounts for about 70 per cent of cases and is characterized by sores that rupture, leaving a yellow-brown crust. Bullous impetigo exhibits large fluid-filled blisters that are painless.

- *Risk factors*: It is most common in pre-school children and highly contagious. It is also common in patients with skin conditions such as scabies, nappy rash, dermatitis or eczema.

- *Causes*: Most cases are caused by *Staphylococcus aureus* that invade the skin through an open wound such as cut or bite. Bacteria penetrate the skin and cause and establish an infection. When the blisters produce fluid, this indicates they are still infectious.

- *Symptoms*: Lesions commonly occur on the face and begin as small vesicles which rapidly enlarge and rupture to form yellow-brown crusts. Underneath this characteristic crust, the lesion is red and moist and may exude fluid. Additional vesicles develop around the primary site and itching is common.

- *Diagnosis and treatment*: Diagnosis is usually by observing symptoms and excluding other skin conditions such as cellulitis, scabies and chickenpox. If the infection does not respond to treatment, a sample may be taken to exclude other conditions. Topical antibiotics may be used on clean, dry skin using gloves to prevent spread of infection. Oral antibiotics may be prescribed for a severe or rapidly spreading infection. With treatment, the infection usually clears within a week. Since it is contagious, infected children should be kept out of school/nursery; towels should not be shared and should be laundered after each use until infection has cleared.

- *Complications*: Although rare, cellulitis can develop which can lead to septicaemia.

33 Eczema   **D. inflammation**

- *Pathophysiology*: Eczema is a form of the inflammatory skin condition dermatitis that causes inflammation of the papillary layer. There are a number of different types but the most common is atopic eczema that mainly affects children and is associated with hypersensitivity reactions.

- *Risk factors*: Atopic eczema tends to be inherited and is associated with allergies, although it tends to disappear as the child gets older.

- *Causes*: As with all forms of dermatitis, the causes and triggers vary between patients. Common triggers include detergents, pet hair and certain foods such as dairy products.

- *Symptoms*: Dry, flaky skin that is sometimes itchy. During a flare-up, symptoms worsen, the skin can become hot (due to the inflammatory reaction) and may ooze or weep, which can become infected.

- *Diagnosis and treatment*: There are no formal diagnostic tests; diagnosis is usually made by examining the symptoms and taking a thorough history of known allergens and any similar family history. Treatment is usually aimed at preventing flare-ups by avoiding known triggers. Emollient creams can be prescribed to moisten skin. During a flare-up corticosteroids may be prescribed to reduce inflammation and an antibiotic may be required for any infection.

FACULTY OF HEALTH + SOCIAL CARE
Library
17 APR 2013
Clatterbridge
UNIVERSITY OF CHESTER

4 The musculoskeletal system

INTRODUCTION

The musculoskeletal system provides structure and support to the body, allowing it to move. It consists of bones, muscle, joints, cartilage, tendons and ligaments. There are three major types of muscle: smooth, skeletal and cardiac muscle. However, only skeletal muscle is involved with movement of the skeleton. There are five types of bone, classified by shape and location, which perform physiological and mechanical functions.

Some diseases and disorders of the musculoskeletal system have a very gradual onset – such as the autoimmune disorder rheumatoid arthritis – while others can be acute – such as fractures. With a gradual onset, patients may have no apparent symptoms for many years, yet damage may be occurring. Most diseases or disorders of this system are diagnosed through X-ray or other bone scans such as computerized tomography (CT), magnetic resonance imaging (MRI) or bone density scanning. With fractures, it is important not to exacerbate the break, ideally patients should not be moved until the limb is splinted.

Many musculoskeletal conditions are chronic and treatment involves controlling symptoms and slowing progression. In fractures, it is important to align and immobilize the broken bone quickly so that healing can begin.

Nurses should appreciate the essential role of the musculoskeletal system in controlling the internal and external movements of the body. It is important to remember that the anatomy and physiology of the musculoskeletal system are influenced by other systems and that disorders of these can affect the body's muscles and skeleton.

Useful resources

Nurses! Test Yourself in Anatomy and Physiology

Chapter 4

Ross and Wilson's Anatomy and Physiology in Health and Illness (11th edition)

Chapter 16

National Institute of Arthritis, Musculoskeletal and Skin Diseases

http://www.niams.nih.gov

LABELLING EXERCISE

1–9 Identify the different kinds of fractures in Figure 4.1, using the terms provided on p. 57.

Figure 4.1 Fracture types

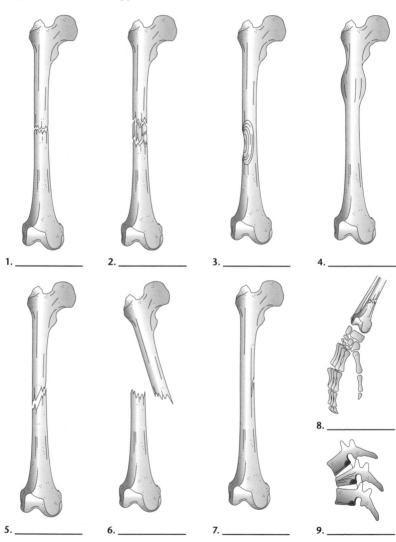

1. _____

2. _____

3. _____

4. _____

5. _____

6. _____

7. _____

8. _____

9. _____

comminuted   compound

crush   pathological

greenstick   spiral

impacted   buckle

simple

TRUE OR FALSE?

Are the following statements true or false?

10   Osteoarthritis is triggered by acute inflammation.

11   Osteoarthritis can be cured with non-steroidal anti-inflammatory drugs.

12   Osteoporosis is a metabolic disease of the skeleton characterized by reduction in bone density.

13   A longitudinal fracture is a break across the diameter of the bone.

14   A person with a suspected fracture may look pale and clammy and feel faint, dizzy or sick.

15   Tendonitis describes inflammation of a tendon.

16   Strain is the injury caused to a bone by overexertion or overuse.

a b c d MULTIPLE CHOICE

Identify one correct answer for each of the following.

17 Which of the following does not contribute to carpal tunnel syndrome?

a) rheumatoid arthritis

b) renal failure

c) heart failure

d) diabetes mellitus

18 Which of the following drugs are used in treating carpal tunnel syndrome?

a) aspirin

b) non-steroidal anti-inflammatory

c) paracetamol

d) morphine

19 Which of the following is not considered an initial symptom of osteoarthritis?

a) muscle wasting

b) pain

c) joint stiffness after wakening

d) limited movement in affected joints

20 Which of the following is often the first specific symptom of osteoporosis?

a) joint pain

b) limb stiffness

c) nerve pain

d) unexplained fracture

21 Osteoporosis usually affects who?

a) children

b) pregnant women

c) older males

d) post-menopausal females

22 Which of the following tests is used to diagnose osteoporosis?

a) X-ray

b) CT scan

c) bone density scan

d) MRI scan

23 What type of fracture describes a bone that does not completely break?

a) compression fracture

b) hairline fracture

c) stress fracture

d) fracture dislocation

24 The most common method of immobilization of a fractured bone is:

a) metal rods

b) pins or screws

c) plaster casts

d) external fixators outside the body

25 Which of the following tests is most commonly used to confirm a fracture?

a) X-ray

b) CT scan

c) bone density scan

d) MRI scan

26 Which of the following is not a symptom of tendonitis?

a) swelling

b) pain and weakness

c) grating or crackling sensation

d) bruising

FILL IN THE BLANKS

Fill in the blanks in each statement using the options in this box.
Not all of them are required, so choose carefully!

calcium	magnesium
multiple sclerosis (MS)	X-rayed
genetic	aligned
carpal tunnel syndrome	muscular dystrophy (MD)
hernia	

27 The most common form of nerve entrapment conditions is _____ _____ _____.

28 A _____ occurs when an internal part of the body, such as an organ, pushes through a weakness in the muscle or surrounding tissue wall.

29 _____ _____ describes a group of inherited diseases characterized by progressive degeneration of groups of muscles.

30 Approximately 40–60 per cent of patients with osteoarthritis will have a _____ link.

31 In addition to bisphosphonate drugs, a _____ supplement may be prescribed if bone density is low.

32 To treat fractures, the broken bones must first be _____; this is known as 'reducing' the fracture.

ANSWERS

 LABELLING EXERCISE

Figure 4.2 Fracture types

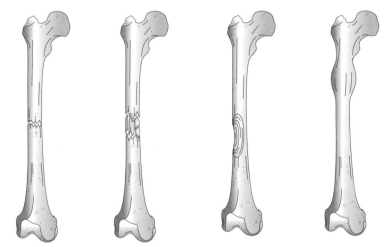

1. Simple fracture 2. Comminuted fracture 3. Pathological fracture 4. Buckle fracture

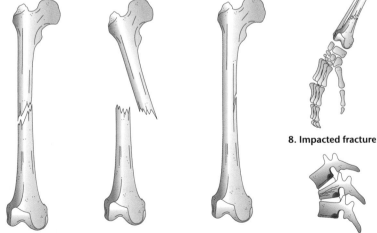

5. Spiral fracture 6. Compound fracture 7. Greenstick fracture

8. Impacted fracture

9. Crush fracture

1 **Simple (closed) fracture:** a clean break where the bone is broken in one place and does not damage surrounding tissue or penetrate the skin.

2 **Comminuted fracture:** the bone shatters into pieces. This type of splinter fracture is difficult to heal and occurs more commonly in serious accidents, such as a depressed fracture of the skull, where the fragment is pushed into the brain.

3 **Pathological fracture:** can occur in a bone weakened by a disease, such as osteoporosis, or by a tumour or cyst.

4 **Buckle (torus) fracture:** occurs commonly in children when the bone deforms but does not crack. It is painful but stable and tends to heal more quickly than greenstick factures.

5 **Spiral fracture:** caused by a twisting motion which results in a winding or slanting break. An oblique fracture (not pictured) is a diagonal fracture of the shaft along the bone's long axis, usually caused by a high impact.

6 **Compound (open) fracture:** occurs when the fractured bone pieces penetrate the skin, damaging surrounding soft tissue. Since the skin is broken there is a higher risk of infection, meaning this kind of fracture is more serious.

7 **Greenstick fracture:** occurs when the bone partly fractures on one side but does not break completely (an incomplete fracture). These are common in children because the young bone is softer, more elastic and able to bend. Greenstick fractures take longer to heal than buckle fractures because they tend to occur in the middle of the bone which is slower growing.

8 **Impacted fracture:** fragments of bone are driven into each other (such as a Colles' fracture of the wrist, pictured).

9 **Crush (compression) fracture:** occurs when the bone collapses. It usually happens in the spongy bone of the spine.

 TRUE OR FALSE?

10 **Osteoarthritis is triggered by acute inflammation.**

Osteoarthritis is the most common form of arthritis and is a chronic condition that damages the hyaline (articular) cartilage in joints, causing secondary damage to the bone, namely development of bony growths and inflammation at the joints. The most commonly affected joints are the knees, hips and small bones in the hands, although any joint may be affected. The degree of disability depends on the site and severity of the cartilage deterioration.

11 **Osteoarthritis can be cured with non-steroidal anti-inflammatory drugs.**

Osteoarthritis is a chronic and incurable condition but symptoms can be managed with painkillers, physiotherapy and surgery where necessary. Patients may also be advised to lose weight where appropriate. There can also be variation between extent of joint damage and severity of symptoms. For example, a joint may be severely damaged without causing symptoms, or symptoms may be severe without affecting movement of the joint.

12 **Osteoporosis is a metabolic disease of the skeleton characterized by reduction in bone density.**

Bone is a living tissue that is constantly growing and replacing itself. As the body ages, a certain amount of bone is lost, causing them to become thinner. Thin bones become fragile and more likely to fracture, particularly the bones of the spine, wrist and hips. Osteoporosis happens more commonly in old age when the body becomes less able to replace worn-out bone. It develops slowly with symptoms appearing gradually; early symptoms include pain or difficulty standing/sitting straight (giving the stooping characteristic).

13 **A longitudinal fracture is a break across the diameter of the bone.**

Longitudinal fractures occur along the length of the bone, transverse fractures break across the bone. An oblique fracture is a diagonal fracture of the shaft along the bone's long axis, usually caused by a high impact.

14 **A person with a suspected fracture may look pale and clammy and feel faint, dizzy or sick.**

This is usually due to pain but may also be due to internal bleeding caused by the fractured bone, particularly large bones such as femur or pelvis. Other symptoms of a fracture include swelling or bruising around the site, the limb may be positioned at an unusual angle, the patient may not be able to weight-bear on the limb or may feel a grinding sensation around the bone. With an open fracture, bleeding will be evident. Irrespective of the type of fracture and where possible, the patient should not be moved until the limb has been immobilized with a splint to prevent movement above and below the fracture site.

15 **Tendonitis describes inflammation of a tendon.**

Tendonitis is inflammation (swelling) of a tendon that causes pain in the affected area. It particularly affects the tendons around the shoulder (suprastinatus tendonitis), elbow (tennis elbow), wrist, finger, thigh, knee or back of the heel (Achilles tendonitis). It is usually caused by overuse of the affected tendon, making it a common sports-related injury, although it can affect anyone. Older adults are also at risk of tendonitis because tendons lose elasticity, becoming weaker over time. Sometimes the sheath around the tendon (rather than the actual tendon) becomes inflamed, this is called tenosynovitis. Tendonitis and tenosynovitis can occur simultaneously.

16 **Strain is the injury caused to a bone by overexertion or overuse.**

Strain is an injury caused to muscle fibres that stretch or tear due to over-use or over-exertion, a common example being hamstring strain. Strains can be prevented by warming-up before exercising. Sprains occur when one or more ligaments are stretched, twisted or torn, usually as a result of excessive force being applied to a joint. Sprains commonly occur at the knee, ankle and wrist. Mild and moderate strains and sprains are usually treated by following the PRICE procedure:

P = prevention by warming-up.
R = resting the muscle after injury.
I = apply an ice pack in short bursts to reduce inflammation.
C = compression with elastic strapping to reduce swelling and inflammation.
E = keep the limb elevated to minimize pain and swelling.

Most people recover normal function 6–8 weeks after a sprain. However, the outlook for strains depends on the severity of the injury and in very severe cases (such as in professional sportspeople) may require surgery.

 MULTIPLE CHOICE

Correct answers identified in bold italics

17 **Which of the following does not contribute to carpal tunnel syndrome?**

a) rheumatoid arthritis   b) renal failure   *c) heart failure*
d) diabetes mellitus

The tendon that passes through the carpal tunnel may become inflamed or fibrous. This causes oedema and compression of the median nerve that runs from the forearm into the hand. Many other conditions which tend to cause fluid retention may also cause swelling in the carpal tunnel, including pregnancy, menopause, hypothyroidism, tuberculosis and benign tumours, as well as oedema due to a bad sprain, dislocation or fracture of the wrist. Symptoms of carpal tunnel syndrome are usually worse at night and in the morning and include pain, burning and paraesthesia (tingling or numbness). Often patients cannot clench the hand in a fist and skin may be dry and shiny. Pain may spread into the forearm and up into the shoulder which can sometimes be relieved by shaking the arm vigorously or hanging the arm down the side.

18 **Which of the following drugs are used in treating carpal tunnel syndrome?**

a) aspirin *b) non-steroidal anti-inflammatory*
c) paracetamol   d) morphine

These drugs reduce inflammation around the median nerve which relieves symptoms. Initially the hand should be rested for 1–2 weeks by splinting the wrist at a neutral angle. If the symptoms are occupation-related, suitable alterations should be made (where possible) to alleviate symptoms. Steroids (cortisone) may be injected into the carpal tunnel to reduce swelling and inflammation around the nerve. Surgical decompression of the median nerve is the last alternative after conservative treatment fails.

19 **Which of the following is not considered an initial symptom of osteoarthritis?**

a) muscle wasting   b) pain   c) joint stiffness after wakening
d) limited movement in affected joints

Pain, limited movement and stiffness in moving are considered the main initial symptoms of osteoarthritis and often develop slowly. Other symptoms may develop as the condition progresses, these include: weakness and muscle wasting, nodules developing on the joints, joint tenderness, a grating sensation when moving the joint and warmth around the joint – indicating inflammation.

20 **Which of the following is often the first specific symptom of osteoporosis?**

a) joint pain   b) limb stiffness   c) nerve pain   *d) unexplained fracture*

A sudden, unexplained fracture may be caused by a simple bump or slight fall that would not cause injury in the absence of osteoporosis. Even a cough or a sneeze may cause a rib fracture. Fractured bones in older people can be serious because the bone is no longer able to repair itself effectively, meaning the patient may have a lasting disability which hinders their independence.

21 **Osteoporosis usually affects who?**

a) children   b) pregnant women   c) older males
d) post-menopausal females

Osteoporosis is related to the decrease in the hormone oestrogen following the menopause. Oestrogen and testosterone are important hormones for processing calcium which is essential for bone formation. Males continue to produce testosterone into old age so osteoporosis is not a big risk for older males. Diseases arising in hormone-producing glands, such as diabetes or hypothyroidism, can leave patients at greater risk of osteoporosis.

22 **Which of the following tests is used to diagnose osteoporosis?**

a) X-ray   b) CT scan   *c) bone density scan*   d) MRI scan

This is the most accurate measurement of bone density and is used to diagnose osteoporosis. A bone density (dual energy X-ray absorptiometry, DEXA) scan measures the density of bones and compares it to a normal range based on the patient's age and gender. The difference between the patient's bone density and the average is calculated and given a 'T score'. A 'T score' between 0 and 1 = normal; −1 and −2.5 = osteopenia – this indicates the bone density between normal and osteoporosis; osteoporosis is only diagnosed if the 'T score' is below −2.5.

23 **What type of fracture describes a bone that does not completely break?**

a) compression fracture   *b) hairline fracture*   c) stress fracture
d) fracture dislocation

This can happen after a trip or fall and can be difficult to detect because the bone is only partially fractured. Stress fractures happen when a bone breaks due to repeated stresses and strains. It is a common complaint in athletes who experience stress fractures in the lower leg or foot bones. Fracture dislocation occurs when the fracture of one of the bones of a joint is accompanied by a dislocation of the same joint. (Avulsion fractures occur when supporting muscle or ligament pulls on the bone, causing it to fracture.)

24 **The most common method of immobilization of a fractured bone is:**

a) metal rods   b) pins or screws   *c) plaster casts*
d) external fixators outside the body

Immobilization is most commonly achieved by encasing the limb in a plaster cast or a brace. In more serious cases, surgery may be required to insert metal pins, plates or screws for immobilization; these require smaller incisions and so are cosmetically more desirable. Internal steel rods immobilize long bones through their centre. In children, flexible wires can be used in the same way. In more serious breaks, external fixators are used to immobilize the bone during healing. These are steel pins that pass into the bone directly through the skin, in order to hold the bones in place. External fixators resemble scaffolding outside the body.

25 **Which of the following tests is most commonly used to confirm a fracture?**

a) X-ray   b) CT scan   c) bone density scan   d) MRI scan

If the fracture is more complex (such as comminuted), then further investigations may be made using CT or MRI scanning. Bone density scanning is not useful when investigating fractures because it measures the amount of calcium in the bones. It can be useful in identifying people who are at greater risk of fractures due to low bone density, such as post-menopausal women who have osteoporosis.

26 **Which of the following is not a symptom of tendonitis?**

a) swelling   b) pain and weakness   c) grating or crackling sensation
d) bruising

Symptoms of tendonitis include pain that becomes worse when moving the affected area. This may be accompanied by weakness, a grating or crackling as the tendon moves, swelling, or a lump may develop along the tendon. Treatment usually involves a period of rest (often with a splint to restrict movement). If symptoms persist, a steroid injection around the affected area may be recommended to reduce inflammation.

FILL IN THE BLANKS

27 **The most common form of nerve entrapment conditions is _carpal tunnel syndrome_.**

Carpal tunnel syndrome (CTS) is a repetitive strain injury resulting from repetitive hand movements that are often occupation-related. It is caused by repeated compression of the median nerve at the wrist. The median nerve is located within the carpal tunnel along with blood vessels and flexor tendons to the fingers and thumb. It is often associated with prolonged keyboard activities such as word-processing. Flexing the wrist is a diagnostic test for carpal tunnel syndrome. If this test produces pain, numbness or tingling, it is likely due to CTS. This test is commonly used in addition to tapping the wrist lightly to see if it produces a tingling feeling or numbness. Together these tests would indicate the median nerve is being compressed and a positive diagnosis of CTS would be made.

28 **A _hernia_ occurs when an internal part of the body, such as an organ, pushes through a weakness in the muscle or surrounding tissue wall.**

A hernia develops when an organ protrudes abnormally through an opening in a muscular wall. The most common types of hernias are: inguinal, femoral and diaphragmatic. An inguinal hernia occurs when part of the bowel protrudes through the lower abdomen into the groin. It is common among males and people who lift heavy weights, but may also be caused by the physical strain associated with persistent cough or chronic constipation. Femoral hernias occur when fatty tissue or a part of the bowel protrudes into the groin. It is less common than inguinal hernias and more common in females. Hiatus hernia (a form of diaphragmatic hernia) occurs when part of the stomach pushes up into the mediastinum of the chest by squeezing through the oesophageal opening in the diaphragm. It is relatively common and sometimes asymptomatic, although a frequent symptom is heartburn. If a hernia is untreated, it may cause serious complications such as bowel obstruction (depending on location) or it can disrupt blood supply to the surrounding herniated tissue (strangulated hernia). Hernias will not disappear without treatment and due to the risk of these potential complications, they are usually surgically repaired.

29 *Muscular dystrophy (MD)* **describes a group of inherited diseases characterized by progressive degeneration of groups of muscles.**

Duchenne muscular dystrophy is the most common form of the condition. It is usually diagnosed around the age of 3 and generally affects males. Symptoms start in the leg muscles, but quickly advance to other muscle groups. Muscles become progressively weaker and the patient usually dies before the age of 30, often due to cardiac or respiratory failure, when the disorder affects intercostal muscles and/or the diaphragm. Another type of MD is Becker muscular dystrophy, the symptoms of which are similar to those of Duchenne MD. However, they are milder and do not usually appear until a person is 10 or 11 years old, or older. Becker MD progresses more slowly than Duchenne MD and patients usually live a normal lifespan. MD is caused by mutations in the genes for healthy muscle structure and function, causing muscle weakness and progressive disability. The different types of MD are caused by mutations in different genes. Not all types of MD cause severe disability, but there is currently no cure for these conditions.

30 **Approximately 40–60 per cent of patients with osteoarthritis will have a *genetic* link.**

Many patients with hand, hip and knee osteoarthritis report family members who have similar symptoms. No gene has yet been identified for the condition. Other risk factors include obesity and previous joint injury. Obesity puts excessive strain on weight-bearing joints while inadequate healing time after injury or surgery to the joint may also be a contributing factor. People who are at risk of osteoarthritis are encouraged to undertake low-impact weight-bearing exercise such as walking (but not jogging) to strengthen bones. (High-impact exercises like jogging could cause weak bones to break.)

31 **In addition to bisphosphonate drugs, a *calcium* supplement may be prescribed if bone density is low.**

A diet rich in calcium (at least 700 mg daily) is recommended to reduce risk of osteoporosis and bone fracture. Patients who are diagnosed with osteoporosis may be prescribed a number of different types of drugs – hormonal and non-hormonal. Previously, hormone replacement therapy (HRT) was prescribed to increase oestrogen levels and therefore enhance calcium absorption but the adverse side effects associated with prolonged HRT now make it a less popular treatment. Bisphosphonates are non-hormonal drugs which maintain bone density and reduce fracture rates.

Osteoporosis patients are usually recommended to take weight-bearing exercise which helps increase bone density.

32 | **To treat fractures, the broken bones must first be *aligned*; this is known as 'reducing' the fracture.**

Aligning the bones brings the broken ends together to allow healing. Once correctly aligned, the ends of the broken bone must be held in position, immobilizing the bone while it heals.

5 The nervous system and special senses

INTRODUCTION

The nervous system is made up of the central and peripheral nervous systems. Together they work to receive, integrate and initiate response to stimuli from inside and outside the body.

Nervous system disorders may be acute or chronic in nature. Many acute conditions can be life-threatening if not diagnosed and treated quickly. Chronic disorders, such as Huntingdon's disease, are frequently irreversible and life-limiting.

Neurological assessment skills are essential in nursing, particularly assessment of consciousness using the Glasgow Coma Scale (GCS). This measures how severely damaged the brain is based on a patient's verbal responses, physical reflexes and how easily they can open their eyes. The highest score is 15, meaning a patient knows where they are and can speak and move as instructed.

With chronic life-limiting neurological disorders, patients are normally prescribed neuro-protective drugs that slow neuro-degeneration. Alongside drug therapy, these patients require social support to help them maintain good quality of life and independence for as long as possible.

Nurses should appreciate how nervous system disorders can have serious and sometimes devastating and degenerative consequences for many organ systems because of its pivotal role in providing communication between the body's organs and systems.

Useful resources

Nurses! Test Yourself in Anatomy and Physiology

Chapter 5

Ross and Wilson's Anatomy and Physiology in Health and Illness (11th edition)

Chapters 7 and 8

Symptoms, Diagnosis and Treatment

Chapters 2 and 3

TRUE OR FALSE?

Are the following statements true or false?

1 Alzheimer's disease is a progressive, degenerative disorder of the cerebrospinal fluid.

2 Epilepsy is triggered by abnormal electrical stimulation of neurones in the brain.

3 Guillain-Barré syndrome is caused by demyelination of central nerves.

4 Induced hypertension is neuroprotective.

5 Hypothermia is neuroprotective because it reduces cerebral oxygen demand.

6 Elevated serum glucose is neuroprotective.

7 In demyelinating conditions neural conduction rates are often increased.

8 A red rash that disappears when a glass is applied is a simple diagnostic test for meningitis.

9 Multiple sclerosis is caused by progressive demyelination of the axons of neurones.

10 Multiple sclerosis patients frequently report the same two initial symptoms.

11 Myasthenia gravis is a neurodegenerative condition characterized by involuntary tremors, progressive muscle rigidity and loss of movement.

12 Stroke occurs when the circulation to the heart is suddenly impaired.

13 The most common cause of problems with the sensory organs is inability to detect stimuli.

MULTIPLE CHOICE

Identify one correct answer for each of the following.

14 Cerebrospinal fluid helps maintain constant:

a) arterial blood pressure

b) venous blood pressure

c) intracranial pressure

d) thoracic pressure

15 Which of the following tests is not used to diagnose Guillain-Barré syndrome?

a) an electrocardiogram (ECG)

b) analysis of protein levels in the cerebrospinal fluid

c) electrophysiology studies

d) electromyography

16 Meningitis causes inflammation of which part of the brain and spinal cord?

a) white matter

b) neurones

c) grey matter

d) meninges

17 The main treatment for bacterial meningitis is usually:

a) no drugs, just rest and fluids

b) paracetamol, rest and fluids

c) antibiotics, rest and fluids

d) antihistamines, rest and fluids

18 The most useful tool for diagnosing multiple sclerosis is:

a) a CT scan

b) an MRI scan

c) blood tests

d) an EEG

19 The main symptoms of Parkinson's disease are:

a) sensory symptoms

b) motor symptoms

c) dementia symptoms

d) immunological symptoms

20 Treatment for Parkinson's disease is mainly aimed at:

a) reversing symptoms

b) relieving symptoms

c) stimulating dopamine production

d) stimulating motor cortex

21 Which of the following is considered a stroke warning?

a) chronic obstructive pulmonary disorder (COPD)

b) deep-vein thrombosis (DVT)

c) myocardial infarction (MI)

d) transient ischaemic attack (TIA)

22 Which system has been introduced and publicized to increase recognition of stroke signs and symptoms?

a) BACK

b) FACE

c) FAST

d) SLOW

23 A head trauma can cause what type of eye injury?

a) retinal detachment

b) cataract

c) glaucoma

d) macular degeneration

24 Which of the following is the most common cause of a perforated eardrum?

a) changes in air pressure

b) middle ear infections

c) loud noise

d) mechanical injury

FILL IN THE BLANKS

Fill in the blanks in each statement using the options in this box.
Not all of them are required, so choose carefully!

Huntingdon's	symptoms
brain	dysaesthesia
vertigo	Fragile X
clot-busting	Parkinson's
lumbar puncture	ultrasound
Guillain-Barré	complications

25 The main symptom of _____-_____ syndrome is progressive ascending muscle weakness and paralysis.

26 A _____ _____ detects elevated pressure in cerebrospinal fluid.

27 A diagnosis of _____ disease is based on the patient's age, history and signs/symptoms rather than laboratory tests.

28 A _____ scan is used to confirm diagnosis of a stroke.

29 When an ischaemic stroke is quickly diagnosed, patients can be treated with _____-_____ drugs.

30 Headache, muscle weakness and paraesthesia are _____ that are common to many nervous system disorders.

31 _____ disease is an incurable, inherited disease that causes gradual deterioration and loss of brain function.

32 _____ describes an inappropriate sense of motion.

ANSWERS

TRUE OR FALSE?

1 **Alzheimer's disease is a progressive, degenerative disorder of the cerebrospinal fluid.**

Alzheimer's disease is a disorder of the cerebral cortex. It is progressive and neurodegenerative. It is a form of dementia and accounts for half of all dementia cases. Degeneration (atrophy) is most notable in the frontal lobes but atrophy occurs in all areas of the cortex with clumps of protein (plaques) forming in the brain as nerve cells become damaged. The exact cause of Alzheimer's disease in unknown although age is the greatest risk factor with majority of patients being over 65 years old. A family history presents only a slightly higher risk although symptoms may present earlier. People with Down's syndrome have a higher risk of developing Alzheimer's disease. Symptoms vary with the severity and progression of the disease but include forgetfulness, irritability, mood swings, incontinence, delusions and obsessive/repetitive behaviour. Although there is no cure, medication (acetylcholinesterase inhibitors which prevent chemical breakdown in the brain) may be prescribed to slow the progression of the disease. Other treatments include establishing appropriate care and support for patients and their carers.

2 **Epilepsy is triggered by abnormal electrical stimulation of neurones in the brain.**

Neurones in the brain are hyper-stimulated, resulting in an excessive amount of electrical activity. This may trigger convulsive movements, of which there are a number of different types. The cerebral cortex is the region of the brain that triggers epileptic seizures. The specific area where the seizure occurs (the epileptogenic focus) varies and is determined by observing the symptoms that occur during a seizure.

3 **Guillain-Barré syndrome is caused by demyelination of central nerves.**

Peripheral nerves are demyelinated in Guillain-Barré syndrome which is sometimes called acute demyelinating polyneuropathy. It is a cell-mediated, autoimmune disorder that is rapidly progressive and potentially fatal, although patients can make a full recovery. Its precise cause is unknown although it often occurs in patients who have recently had influenza (viral infection) or respiratory disorders. There are three clinical phases in the syndrome. The acute phase, when symptoms first develop, lasts 1–3 weeks and ends when no further deterioration is observed. The plateau phase is the second phase and can last from a few days to two weeks. The recovery phase lasts longest. It is thought to correspond with remyelination and can last from four months to three years. Recovery is not always complete and patients often need rehabilitation assistance in the form of occupational therapy and physiotherapy.

4 | **Induced hypertension is neuroprotective.**

This is part of controlled triple 'H' therapy: <u>h</u>ypertension to increase perfusion; <u>h</u>aemodilution to increase plasma volume and pressure; and <u>h</u>ypervolaemia to do both. This procedure can be used to treat vasospasm (a serious complication of subarachnoid haemorrhage (SAH)), its aim is to keep the blood vessels open (haemodilution and hypervolaemia) and the tissue perfused (hypertension), to prevent ischaemia in the brain.

5 | **Hypothermia is neuroprotective because it reduces cerebral oxygen demand.**

There is a 50 per cent reduction in oxygen demand as core body temperature falls from 37°C to 27°C, this happens because hypothermia slows the metabolism which requires oxygen, therefore reducing the risk of ischaemic tissue injury, hence protecting the delicate nervous tissue. This is why transplant organs are stored in ice and it is the basis for therapeutic (induced) hypothermia where the patient's body temperature is reduced under medical supervision. A number of brain injury patients have had a better long-term outcome after this treatment.

6 | **Elevated serum glucose is neuroprotective.**

Elevated levels of plasma glucose (hyperglycaemia) are considered dangerous. They cause a greater-than-expected fall in intracellular pH because excess glucose may produce lactic acid (which lowers blood pH) during ischaemia. Furthermore, glucose-induced arteriolar dilation impairs effective vasoregulation and facilitates hypertensive damage to all organs.

7 | **In demyelinating conditions neural conduction rates are often increased.**

In demyelinating conditions the myelin covering on the axon of the neurone is depleted or reduced. Thinner myelin allows sodium channels to spread out from the nodes, thus slowing conduction rates of the electrical nerve impulse, and saltatory conduction is lost. The most common demyelinating condition is multiple sclerosis (MS). Others include diphtheria which is caused by a bacterial infection of the respiratory tract and Guillain-Barré syndrome which can occur after a viral infection (see Answer 3).

8 | **A red rash that disappears when a glass is applied is a simple diagnostic test for meningitis.**

The red rash should *not* disappear when a glass is gently pressed on the skin. There are many signs and symptoms of meningitis including, headache, stiff neck, aversion to light, fatigue, vomiting, seizures, fever and chills. Infants and children may be fretful or refuse food. Other diagnostic tests include the Brudzinski's sign or Kernig's sign. In Brudzinski's sign, a patient in the dorsal recumbent position (lying on back, head and shoulders) involuntarily flexes the hips and knees when the neck is bent forward. For Kernig's sign, pain or resistance when the hip and knee are flexed in the supine position, indicates meningitis.

9 | **Multiple sclerosis is caused by progressive demyelination of the axons of neurones.**

Demyelination describes the loss or destruction of the myelin sheath covering some nerve fibres which results in their impaired function preventing the normal conduction of the electrical impulses along affected neurones. After myelin is destroyed, a hard plaque of scar tissue forms in its place and disrupts the conduction of nerve impulses. Symptoms of MS are unpredictable and become irreversible as the disease progresses.

10 | **Multiple sclerosis patients frequently report the same two initial symptoms.**

Patients often find it difficult to describe symptoms but a patient history often reveals two initial symptoms, namely visual disturbances and other sensory impairments. After these initial events, symptoms vary and depend on the extent of myelin loss, the site of myelin loss, the extent of any remyelination and the quality of nerve transmission at the synapses after remyelination. Other signs and symptoms include fatigue, muscle weakness, paralysis, poor speech, poor gait, urinary and bowel problems.

11 | **Myasthenia gravis is a neurodegenerative condition characterized by involuntary tremors, progressive muscle rigidity and loss of movement.**

These symptoms are characteristic of the neurodegenerative disorder, Parkinson's disease (PD) which affects movement. In PD, there is a reduction in the amount of the neurotransmitter hormone, dopamine, in the basal ganglia of the brain; this reduces stimulation of the motor cortex in the brain.

Myasthenia gravis is an autoimmune disorder that produces sporadic, progressive weakness and fatigue of voluntary muscles. It is relatively rare and most commonly affects females under 40 years. Antibodies in the immune system attack and damage the nerve signal reception areas on muscles (post-synaptic neuromuscular junction) preventing communication between nerve and muscle; this results in a loss of effectiveness of the muscle.

12 | **Stroke occurs when the circulation to the heart is suddenly impaired.**

Stroke or cerebrovascular accident (CVA) describes a decrease in circulation to the brain. Reduction in circulation to the heart is described as myocardial infarction (MI or heart attack). CVA can occur when the brain is deprived of oxygenated blood, this can happen in two ways:

I. A blood vessel in the brain becomes blocked by a blood clot, this blockage is known as an intracranial or cerebral aneurysm and can lead to an ischaemic stroke.
II. A blood vessel in the brain bursts (usually because of an aneurysm) causing a haemorrhagic stroke.

Both events result in the brain tissue being deprived of oxygen causing necrosis (uncontrolled tissue death) from lack of oxygen and accumulation of toxic carbon dioxide. The majority (70–80 per cent) of strokes are ischaemic events.

13 **The most common cause of problems with the sensory organs is inability to detect stimuli.**

There are three possible problems that can account for disorders of the sensory organs (eyes, ears, nose, tongue and sensory receptors for touch, pressure or temperature):

I. Stimuli cannot be detected by receptors.
II. Receptors do not respond normally to stimuli.
III. Integration and communication pathways are defective.

Detection of stimuli is the main problem associated with sensory disorders; examples include cataracts on the eyes which prevent light from reaching the retina of the eye and conductive deafness where sound is unable to enter the inner ear. Examples of sensory disorders where stimuli reach receptors but receptors do not respond normally include colour blindness, inherited deafness and deafness caused by loud noise. Examples of disorders caused by defects in integration and communication of stimuli include glaucoma or brain damage caused by stroke or other cranial trauma.

 MULTIPLE CHOICE

Correct answers identified in bold italics

14 **Cerebrospinal fluid helps maintain constant:**

a) arterial blood pressure   b) venous blood pressure
c) intracranial pressure   d) thoracic pressure

Intracranial pressure (ICP) is affected by brain size and volume of blood vessels and cerebrospinal fluid (CSF). Sometimes the effects of raised ICP are more serious than the condition causing it. Raised ICP is usually accompanied by hypertension and bradycardia.

15 **Which of the following tests is not used to diagnose Guillain-Barré syndrome?**

a) an electrocardiogram (ECG)   b) analysis of protein levels in the cerebrospinal fluid   c) electrophysiology studies   d) electromyography

All of the other tests can be used in the diagnosis of Guillain-Barré syndrome. ECG records the electrical activity of the heart over time by placing electrodes on the surface of the skin. CSF analysis may indicate normal white blood cell levels but elevated protein levels and in severe cases, increased pressure of CSF. The CSF protein levels will continue to increase and peak around 4–6 weeks after the onset of signs and symptoms, indicating widespread inflammation of nerve roots. Electrophysiology studies may indicate slower conduction of electrical impulses between nerves. Electromyography (EMG) records electrical activity produced by the skeletal muscle cells.

16 **Meningitis causes inflammation of which part of the brain and spinal cord?**

a) white matter   b) neurones   c) grey matter   *d) meninges*

All three membranes of the meninges may be inflamed – dura mater, arachnoid mater and pia mater. The inflammation causes tissues to swell and increases the ICP which reduces blood flow to the brain. Inflammation may be caused by a range of pathogens, but the most common causes of meningitis are bacteria and viruses.

17 **The main treatment for bacterial meningitis is usually:**

a) no drugs, just rest and fluids   b) paracetamol, rest and fluids
c) antibiotics, rest and fluids   d) antihistamines, rest and fluids

Patients with bacterial meningitis will be treated with intravenous (IV) antibiotics when sent to hospital, followed by oral antibiotics along with rest and plenty of fluids. The most common antibiotic prescribed is penicillin but where there is a known allergy, tetracycline, chloramphenicol or kanamycin are used. For viral meningitis, antibiotics are not appropriate. Until a bacterial cause is excluded, patients will be treated with antibiotics which are then withdrawn upon a viral diagnosis. Patients are advised to rest and remain hydrated.

18 **The most useful tool for diagnosing multiple sclerosis is:**

a) a CT scan   *b) an MRI scan*   c) blood tests   d) an EEG

An MRI will detect lesions and also indicate the extent of the disease. Up to 90 per cent of patients will have detectable lesions by the time an MRI is performed. A CT scan will identify lesions in the brain's white matter. White blood cells (WBC) may be elevated while an EEG will identify abnormalities in about one-third of patients.

19 **The main symptoms of Parkinson's disease are:**

a) sensory symptoms   **b) motor symptoms**   c) dementia symptoms
d) immunological symptoms

Since Parkinson's disease (PD) affects the motor cortex of the brain, the first symptoms that patients experience involve motor functions, of which there are four major types:

I.   tremor;
II.   muscle rigidity – due to joint stiffness;
III.   akinesia (slow/impaired muscle movement) or bradykinesia (extremely slow movement);
IV.   unstable posture.

Further symptoms develop including fatigue (due to persistent tremor), dysphagia (difficulty swallowing), impaired speech, increased perspiration, oily skin, insomnia and often depression and mood changes – due to the frustration of the condition. Patients do not suffer from dementia although it can develop later in the condition. Complications include injury due to falls as a consequence of unstable gait, food aspiration due to impaired swallow, urinary tract infections and skin breakdown due to immobility.

20 **Treatment for Parkinson's disease is aimed at:**

a) reversing symptoms   **b) relieving symptoms**
c) stimulating dopamine production   d) stimulating motor cortex

Currently there is no cure for PD or reversal of symptoms. Treatment aims to relieve symptoms and halt progression, maintaining motor function for as long as possible. Drug therapy includes dopamine replacement (but does not stimulate production), however, this can cause adverse effects. Alongside dopamine therapy, patients may receive anticholinergics or antihistamines to reduce tremors. Physiotherapy is also helpful in maintaining muscle function and tone. Deep brain stimulation is a surgical technique to help treat motor symptoms of PD. A tiny electrical pulse (similar to a heart pacemaker) produces a current in the affected area of the brain. Some PD patients have reported a significant improvement in their motor function. The procedure carries a small risk of stroke and the long-term effectiveness of the procedure has yet to be fully assessed.

21 **Which of the following is considered a stroke warning?**

a) chronic obstructive pulmonary disorder (COPD)
b) deep-vein thrombosis (DVT)   c) myocardial infarction (MI)
d) transient ischaemic attack (TIA)

Transient ischaemic attack (TIA or 'mini-stroke') is considered a warning of an impending severe stroke. TIA is a temporary interruption of blood blow, usually in the small distal branches of the brain's arteries, which results in lack of oxygen in the brain. TIAs are thought to be due to small microemboli that break off from a thrombus and temporarily halt blood flow and hence reduce oxygen supply. They are said to be transient because symptoms disappear in less than 24 hours and normal neurological function returns. The signs and symptoms are usually an indicator of the affected artery and include double vision, unilateral blindness, lack of coordination, numbness, dizziness, speech difficulty (FAST symptoms, see Answer 22). Treatment of a TIA aims to prevent a complete stroke by administering aspirin to thin blood or anticoagulants to reduce development of thrombosis. Symptoms lasting longer than 24 hours indicate a 'full' stroke.

22 | **Which system has been introduced and publicized to increase recognition of stroke signs and symptoms?**

a) BACK   b) FACE   *c) FAST – meaning: f̲ace, a̲rm, s̲peech, t̲ime*   d) SLOW

This acronym has been used to raise awareness of stroke symptoms. It indicates the major signs and symptoms of a stroke: facial drooping or paralysis on one side, weakness or paralysis of one or both arms and distorted speech. When any of these symptoms arise in a patient, people are encouraged to immediately seek emergency medical help. The earlier a patient receives treatment for a stroke, the less severe the long-term neurological effects will be. Patients with suspected ischaemic stroke will be immediately treated with a 'clot-busting' (or thrombolytic) medicine called alteplase, which dissolves blood clots. However, alteplase is only effective if used during the first three hours after a stroke has taken place. After an ischaemic stroke, long-term preventative treatment may include aspirin or anticoagulants (such as heparin or warfarin) to thin the blood and reduce the risk of further clots developing. In haemorrhagic stroke patients, emergency surgery on the skull (craniotomy) is often required to remove any blood from the brain and repair any burst blood vessels. Blood pressure- and/or cholesterol-modifying medications may also be necessary long-term treatments after both types of stroke.

23 | **A head trauma can cause what type of eye injury?**

a) retinal detachment   b) cataract   c) glaucoma
d) macular degeneration

A serious head injury can cause the retina to separate from the inner wall of the eye. The most common symptom of retinal detachment is a shadow or 'black curtain' spreading across the vision. Vision may become cloudy as small blood vessels bleed into the vitreous humor of the eye. Symptoms also include floaters in the vision or flashing bright lights. There is no pain with retinal detachment. Risk factors include short-sightedness (because the retina can be thinner) and diabetes. It can occur as a complication of cataract surgery. Surgery to reattach the retina is the only treatment, without which blindness will develop.

Glaucoma is a disease in which the optic nerve is damaged, leading to progressive, irreversible loss of vision. It is often, but not always, associated with increased pressure of the fluid in the eye. Macular degeneration refers to loss of central vision due to denegation of the retina and is the major cause of visual impairment in older adults. Cataracts occur when parts of the lens become cloudy as changes occur in the proteins within the lens. Cataracts reduce the amount of light entering the eye and so vision appears cloudy. They can develop as a complication of diabetes mellitus.

24 **Which of the following is the most common cause of a perforated eardrum?**

a) changes in air pressure   *b) middle ear infections*   c) loud noise
d) mechanical injury

Although all of these situations can cause perforation of the eardrum (tympanic membrane), the most common cause is due to infections of the middle ear. During an ear infection pus can build up inside the ear, putting pressure on the eardrum. With accumulating pressure the eardrum ruptures, allowing the pus to escape. This mucus discharge is a common symptom of a perforated eardrum. Perforated eardrum can sometimes be caused by injury (such as with a cotton bud) or by shock waves from a very loud noise (such as an explosion). Damage from loud noise often causes severe hearing loss and ringing in the ears (tinnitus). Sudden changes in air pressure, such as changes in altitude in an aircraft, often cause pain in the ear. Occasionally, these sudden pressure changes can perforate the eardrum. This occurs because there is a big difference between the air pressure outside the ear and the air pressure inside the middle ear. A perforated eardrum will often heal by itself within 6–8 weeks. Painkillers may be prescribed to ease symptoms and antibiotics may be administered if the ear is infected. If damage is more serious, surgery may be required.

FILL IN THE BLANKS

25 **The main symptom of _Guillain-Barré_ syndrome is progressive ascending muscle weakness and paralysis.**

Symptoms of this condition usually arise after an acute infection. Patients begin to notice symmetrical weakness which usually affects the lower limbs first and rapidly progresses, in an ascending fashion, up the legs. Patients generally notice weakness in their legs or legs that tend to buckle, with or without numbness or tingling (dysaesthesia). As the weakness progresses upward, usually over periods of hours to days, the arms and facial muscles also become affected. Patients are often very distressed and seek medical attention at this stage. Patients must be monitored as the paralysis spreads, since it may become life-threatening if it reaches the respiratory or cardiac muscles. Patients are often admitted to intensive care units.

26 **A _lumbar puncture_ detects elevated pressure in cerebrospinal fluid.**

Lumbar puncture (LP or spinal tap) involves inserting a needle into the spinal canal to extract a sample of cerebrospinal fluid (CSF), which is then examined in a laboratory. The CSF may be a cloudy or milky colour, protein levels may be elevated and glucose concentration decreased. LP can be used to diagnose meningitis and a positive Gram stain can assist in identifying the infecting bacteria. A chest X-ray can identify pneumonia, lung abscess or lesions causing fungal meningitis. A CT scan is usually performed before LP to exclude cerebral haemorrhage, haematoma or tumour that may cause meningitis because performing LP on such patients can be dangerous. LP can sometimes be used to administer antibiotics or chemotherapy and although rare, LP may be used to remove excess CSF and relieve high ICP which can develop in rare conditions such as SAH or Lyme disease.

27 **A diagnosis of *Parkinson's* disease is based on the patient's age, history and signs/symptoms rather than laboratory tests.**

Laboratory tests provide little diagnostic information during investigations for PD. However, a urinalysis test may indicate decreased dopamine levels. CT or magnetic resonance imaging (MRI) scans may be used to exclude other disorders, such as a tumour, that could cause similar symptoms. Initial diagnosis is usually made based on symptoms, history and clinical examination. If PD is suspected, the patient would be referred to a specialist such as a neurologist or geriatrician.

28 **A *brain* scan is used to confirm diagnosis of a stroke.**

All patients with suspected stroke should receive a brain scan within 24 hours. A brain scan will determine the type of stroke (ischaemic or haemorrhagic) and therefore the type of treatment. Some treatments need to be given quickly, so rapid access to diagnostic tests is important. Therefore, if a person is suspected of having a severe stroke, a CT scan is sufficient to identify the region of the stroke and whether it is due to bleeding or a clot. Since a CT scanning is quicker than an MRI, this speeds up the diagnostic time meaning thrombolysis ('clot-busting') treatment can be administered more quickly, which is essential when treating stroke patients. An MRI scan is more appropriate if symptoms are complicated or when the extent or location of the stroke is unclear. The MRI provides more detail of cerebral tissue, allowing smaller strokes to be identified or TIAs which occur in unusual locations.

29 **When an ischaemic stroke is quickly diagnosed, patients can be treated with *clot-busting* drugs.**

Ischaemic strokes are caused by clots. Clot-busting (thrombolysis) treatment with alteplase is only effective if administered within a few hours of symptoms developing. The treatment breaks down clots, allowing blood to flow normally. This treatment is not used for patients with haemorrhagic strokes, since it thins the blood and enhances bleeding. Antiplatelet medicines, such as aspirin, reduce the likelihood of future blood clots but again are not advisable as treatment for haemorrhagic strokes. Anticoagulant therapy with heparin or warfarin is recommended for many people with TIA or stroke who have an irregular heartbeat (atrial fibrillation) but not for haemorrhagic strokes. Haemorrhagic stroke patients may have emergency cranial surgery (craniotomy) to reduce ICP and should have blood pressure, blood glucose and oxygen levels monitored. Long-term treatment focuses on lowering blood pressure with angiotensin-converting enzyme (ACE) inhibitor drugs, which widen the blood vessels and reduce blood pressure. Physical and psychological rehabilitation after a serious stroke involves long-term lifestyle changes with many patients developing depression due to their lack of independence after a severe stroke.

30 **Headache, muscle weakness and paraesthesia are *symptoms* that are common to many nervous system disorders.**

Symptoms of nervous system disorders can be diverse although headache, muscle weakness and paraesthesia (numbness or tingling) accompany many disorders of this system. Headaches are usually due to muscle tension. Muscle weakness can be caused by muscle diseases (myopathies) or neurological diseases (such as demyelinating diseases) and it is essential that the underlying cause of muscle weakness is determined for accurate diagnosis and treatment. Paraesthesia may be temporary or permanent.

31 ***Huntingdon's* disease is an incurable, inherited disease that causes gradual deterioration and loss of brain function.**

Although rare, Huntingdon's disease has devastating consequences for the families it affects. The major symptom involves a decline in motor, cognitive and behavioural functions which are usually first observed in early adulthood (between 20 and 35 years old). These progressively decline, leading to dementia and death (although death is usually due to a secondary cause such as heart failure, pneumonia or other infection). As symptoms progress, the patient needs increasing nursing care, particularly in the later stages of the disease. Diagnosis is by genetic testing for the faulty gene, although nowadays families that carry the defective gene would probably be aware of their risk before symptoms develop. No treatment currently exists and progression cannot be slowed. Speech and occupational therapy are recommended while many patients will be prescribed medication to control involuntary tremors and some require antidepressants to treat mood swings and depression.

32 ***Vertigo* describes an inappropriate sense of motion.**

People who experience vertigo report a sensation of movement or spinning even when they are completely still, symptoms also include nausea and loss of balance. It is commonly caused by a problem with the balance mechanisms within the inner ear due to viral infection, although it can also be caused by nerve damage between the middle ear and the brain or by damage to the brain itself. Initial treatment is with an antihistamine such as cyclizine or prochlorperazine – both will alleviate the nausea associated with vertigo. Patients often find relief from symptoms by lying still in a dark, quiet room. Vertigo that reoccurs or persists may be caused by an underlying condition, such as tinnitus or Ménière's disease, and should be investigated.

6 The endocrine system

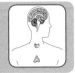

INTRODUCTION

The hypothalamus in the brain is vital for regulating hormones, the chemical messengers of the endocrine system. The other organs of the endocrine system include the adrenal glands, the pancreas, the pituitary gland and the thyroid gland. Feedback systems regulate the endocrine system by controlling the production of hormones.

If a patient has abnormal levels of a hormone circulating in the blood, it may be due to a disorder of the endocrine system caused by abnormal secretion of the hormones, poor response to hormones by their receptor organs or cells, inflammation or a tumour of the hormone-producing gland.

Many endocrine disorders have very general symptoms such as weight loss or gain, fatigue, nausea. Therefore, a detailed patient history and blood tests are usually required to achieve an accurate diagnosis. Patients with an endocrine disorder should be assessed for defects in the gland, problems with release of hormones, transport of hormones or with the effector organ.

Knowing how the endocrine system is responsible for continuous communication and control can help nurses understand how disruption of this system can lead to widespread disorder in the body.

Useful resources

Nurses! Test Yourself in Anatomy and Physiology

Chapter 6

Ross and Wilson's Anatomy and Physiology in Health and Illness (11th edition)

Chapter 9

TRUE OR FALSE?

Are the following statements true or false?

1 In most countries, blood glucose is reported in terms of molarity.

2 Type 2 diabetes mellitus is insulin dependent.

3 Gestational diabetes mellitus occurs during pregnancy.

4 Diabetes insipidus is another name for diabetes mellitus.

5 A 24-hour urinary cortisol test can be used to diagnose Cushing's syndrome.

6 A symptom of hyperthyroidism is increased weight.

7 Graves' disease is a form of hypothyroidism.

8 In hypothyroidism, metabolic processes are suppressed.

MULTIPLE CHOICE

Identify one correct answer for each of the following.

9 Which of the following is a symptom of hypoglycaemia?

a) dehydration

b) palpitations

c) polydypsia

d) polyuria

10 The target of glycaemic control is an HbA1c blood level of:

a) below 42 mmol/mol

b) 45 mmol/mol

c) 48 mmol/mol

d) above 53 mmol/mol

11 Diabetes insipidus is caused by a deficiency in:

a) angiotensin

b) antidiuretic hormone

c) insulin

d) renin

12 Which of these disorders is not related to the thyroid gland?

a) Addison's disease

b) hyperthyroidism

c) hypothyroidism

d) goitre

13 Cushing's syndrome is characterized by an excess of which type of hormone?

a) antidiuretic hormone

b) glucagon

c) glucocorticoids

d) aldosterone

14 Which of the following is not a chronic complication of diabetes mellitus?

a) cardiovascular disease

b) retinopathy

c) kidney disease

d) diabetic ketoacidosis

15 Which of the following is not a symptom of hypothyroidism?

a) fatigue

b) unexplained weight gain

c) diarrhoea

d) sensitivity to cold

FILL IN THE BLANKS

Fill in the blanks in each statement using the options in this box.
Not all of them are required, so choose carefully!

Addison's	hyperthyroidism
hypothyroidism	glucagon
glucose	Parkinson's
Cushing's	

16 Insulin is the main hormone that regulates cellular uptake of _____ from the blood.

17 A patient with _____ disease would exhibit symptoms including weight loss, dehydration and a craving for salty food.

18 A complication of _____ disease is hypertension which can lead to ischaemic heart disease.

19 Radioactive iodine therapy is the primary treatment for_____.

20 Thyroid hormone replacement is used in the treatment of _____.

ANSWERS

TRUE OR FALSE?

1 | **In most countries, blood glucose is reported in terms of molarity.**

In most countries, blood glucose is reported in terms of molarity, measured in millimoles per litre (abbreviated as mmol/L) or millimolar (abbreviated mM). In the USA, blood glucose is reported as mass concentration and measured in mg/dL. To convert blood glucose readings:

Divide the mg/dL figure by 18 (or multiply by 0.055) to get mmol/L.

The measurement reports the concentration of glucose in the blood. It varies with each individual and the time of day but normal blood glucose levels before a meal (pre-prandial) is in the range of 4.0–6.0 mmol/L and less than 10.0 mmol/L two hours after a meal (post-prandial).

2 | **Type 2 diabetes mellitus is insulin dependent.**

Diabetes mellitus (DM) is a chronic condition characterized by excess glucose in the blood. Insulin is a hormone produced by the pancreas that normally regulates the concentration of glucose in the blood. DM can be caused by either:

- insufficient or no insulin being produced; or
- the body is unable to respond to the insulin it produces.

Irrespective of the cause, the end result is the same: the body is unable to use the glucose in the blood for energy which causes hyperglycaemia. The two major types of diabetes mellitus are: type 1 which is insulin dependent (previously known as insulin dependent diabetes mellitus – IDDM) and type 2 which is *not* insulin dependent (previously known as non-insulin dependent diabetes mellitus). Type 1 DM is caused by the autoimmune destruction or abnormal function of beta cells, usually due to a genetic defect; this prevents insufficient insulin being produced. It usually develops early in life, hence it was also previously known as juvenile diabetes.

Type 2 DM is much more common, accounting for over 90 per cent of all cases of DM. In type 2 DM, the body's cells become unresponsive to insulin and therefore are unable to utilize the glucose obtained from dietary carbohydrates; in addition, the beta cells may be gradually destroyed over time which increases insulin resistance in patients. It is strongly associated with obesity and previously occurred more frequently in older individuals. With the increase in obesity in children and young people, more cases of type 2 DM are being diagnosed in younger people. This will have a serious impact on the long-term care and treatment of DM patients who may live with the disease for many decades and will therefore be more at risk of developing complications associated with DM. Initial clinical symptoms of type 2 DM are usually mild and can often be controlled by diet, exercise and weight loss. However, the longer a person lives with the condition, the more severe their symptoms may become, eventually requiring insulin to control blood glucose levels.

3 **Gestational diabetes mellitus occurs during pregnancy.**

The third type of DM is gestational diabetes which only develops during pregnancy and disappears after birth. Gestational diabetes refers to the mother having DM and not the foetus. It is caused by changes to the maternal glucose metabolism during pregnancy. Although the condition may be mild and produce few symptoms in the mother, it presents similar dangers to the foetus as other types of diabetes and often the babies have a high birth weight and are more at risk of jaundice. Mothers who are already diabetic need to be monitored very closely during pregnancy to reduce the risk of complications related to their diabetes. Those who develop gestational diabetes are at greater risk of type 2 DM later in life.

4 **Diabetes insipidus is another name for diabetes mellitus.**

Diabetes insipidus (DI) is not the same as diabetes mellitus (DM). The term 'diabetes' is usually used to describe diabetes mellitus. DI is a rarer form of 'diabetes', considered to be a disorder of the pituitary gland whereas DM is considered a disorder of the pancreas. DI is characterized by excretion of a large volume of urine (polyuria) which is very dilute but does not contain glucose. The volume of urine is not reduced when fluid intake is reduced, indicating the kidneys are unable to concentrate urine. In diabetes mellitus, the excess urine produced is always sweet due to the excess glucose in the urine (glycosuria).

5 **A 24-hour urinary cortisol test can be used to diagnose Cushing's syndrome.**

This test determines the excretion rate of the free steroid hormone cortisol. Increased levels of urinary cortisol would confirm a diagnosis of Cushing's syndrome (see Answer 13). Cortisol levels rise and fall throughout the day with the highest levels usually between 6 a.m. and 8 a.m. and the lowest around midnight. The normal range of urinary cortisol is between 10–100 micrograms per 24 hours.

6 **A symptom of hyperthyroidism is increased weight.**

Hyperthyroidism (over-active thyroid) causes an increase in metabolic processes characterized by decrease in body weight despite an increased appetite. Other signs and symptoms include tremors, palpitations, sweating, diarrhoea, heat intolerance, protrusion of the eyes and enlarged thyroid gland. Weight gain is a symptom of hypothyroidism due to the slowing down of the metabolism.

7 **Graves' disease is a form of hypothyroidism.**

Graves' disease is an autoimmune disorder that causes goitre and is the most common cause of hyperthyroidism. Other causes of hyperthyroidism include a thyroid tumour, pituitary tumour or inflammation of the thyroid gland.

8 **In hypothyroidism, metabolic processes are suppressed.**

Hypothyroidism (under-active thyroid) occurs when levels of thyroid hormones in the blood are low. The slowing down of metabolic processes is caused by the decrease in the levels of the triiodothyronine (T_3) and thyroxine (T_4) hormones that regulate metabolic activity and protein synthesis. The disorder is more common in females and people with Down's syndrome. Primary hypothyroidism indicates a problem with the thyroid gland while secondary hypothyroidism indicates a failure to stimulate normal thyroid function, for example when the pituitary gland does not secrete enough thyroid-stimulating hormone (TSH).

MULTIPLE CHOICE

Correct answers identified in bold italics

9 **Which of the following is a symptom of hypoglycaemia?**

a) dehydration ***b) palpitations*** c) polydypsia d) polyuria

Hypoglycaemia is an acute complication of DM, it indicates a lower than normal level of blood glucose (usually lower than 3.8 mmol/L). The brain tissue and cells are dependent on a continuous supply of glucose from the blood, therefore, if the amount of glucose supplied by the blood falls, the brain is one of the first organs affected. Patients who become hypoglycaemic may exhibit a number of signs and symptoms such as sweating, clamminess, feeling cold, paraesthesia, headache, nausea and vomiting, double vision, slurred speech, irritability, confusion, fatigue, poor coordination (sometimes appearing drunk), seizures and may even lapse into a coma if the condition is not reversed. If conscious, patients may be treated by rapid glucose administration (such as a high glucose drink).

Polydypsia (increased thirst), polyphagia (increased appetite) and polyuria (frequent urination) are the main symptoms of DM. In type 1 DM, such symptoms can develop quickly (even over a few weeks) but in type 2 DM symptoms are more subtle and develop over a much longer time.

10 **The target of glycaemic control is an HbA1c blood level of:**

a) below 42 mmol/mol b) 45 mmol/mol ***c) 48 mmol/mol***
d) above 53 mmol/mol

Glycaemic control is a medical term referring to the average levels of blood glucose in a DM patient. The long-term complications of DM result from many years of hyperglycaemia, so good glycaemic control indicates the condition is quite stable which is an important goal for DM patients to reduce the risk of complications. Glucose in the blood binds to haemoglobin, forming glycosylated haemoglobin called HbA1c. The higher the HbA1c level, the more glucose is present in the blood, which is undesirable as it can accelerate development of complications associated with hyperglycaemia. Measuring HbA1c provides an accurate reading of the blood glucose levels over the previous 2–3 months. Ideally, consecutive readings should be low, under 48mmol/mol, although the exact target is set for individual patients based on their symptoms. Control and outcomes of both types 1 and 2 DM may be improved by patients using home glucose meters to regularly monitor their blood glucose levels. However, these meters only measure the amount of glucose in the blood at the specific time of testing.

11 | **Diabetes insipidus is caused by a deficiency in:**

a) angiotensin   *b) antidiuretic hormone*   c) insulin   d) renin

Diabetes insipidus (DI) is caused by lack of antidiuretic hormone (ADH or vasopressin) production (hyposecretion) or lack of renal response to ADH. Hyposecretion may be caused by damage to the pituitary gland which releases ADH, while lack of renal response may be due to damage to the kidneys, making them insensitive to ADH. DI caused by hyposecretion of ADH can be treated with hormone replacement therapy. However, renal DI due to insensitivity to ADH is more difficult to treat.

12 | **Which of these disorders is not related to the thyroid gland?**

a) Addison's disease   b) hyperthyroidism   c) hypothyroidism
d) goitre

Addison's disease is a disorder of the adrenal glands; it is also known as adrenal hypofunction or adrenal dysfunction. The primary form of Addison's disease originates in the adrenal glands and is characterized by low secretion of the steroid hormones mineralocorticoids (mainly aldosterone), glucocorticoids (mainly cortisol) and androgen. The secondary form may arise from a disorder outside the adrenal glands such as a pituitary tumour. Goitre is an enlargement of the thyroid gland which can be caused by a lack of iodine in the diet or can arise sporadically particularly from certain foods or drugs. Goitre can be classified toxic or non-toxic. Hypothyroidism occurs when the thyroid gland is under-active, producing insufficient amounts of thyroid hormone. Hyperthyroidism is caused by over-production of the thyroid hormone.

13 | **Cushing's syndrome is characterized by an excess of which type of hormone?**

a) antidiuretic hormone   b) glucagon   *c) glucocorticoids*
d) aldosterone

Cushing's syndrome is caused when the adrenal glands secrete excess amounts of the glucocorticoid hormones and sometimes excess androgens as well. In most patients, Cushing's syndrome is the result of an over-secretion of corticotrophin which causes excessive cell proliferation in the adrenal cortex.

14 **Which of the following is not a chronic complication of diabetes mellitus?**

a) cardiovascular disease   b) retinopathy   c) kidney disease
d) diabetic ketoacidosis (DKA)

This is an acute complication of hyperglycaemia, caused by a combination of ketosis (an accumulation of ketones in the blood) and acidosis (increase in acidity of the blood). In DM patients their body cells are unable to take in glucose circulating in the blood and so cells begin to use protein and fats for energy. Fat metabolism causes the accumulation of ketones in the blood. Ketones are toxic, acidic compounds that cause an increase in the acidity of the blood (acidosis), hence lowering the blood pH. Symptoms of DKA include nausea, vomiting, blurred vision, and rapid, deep breathing (as the body attempts to expel the excess ketones). Vomiting can exacerbate the condition by causing dehydration. The breath may smell of acetone or pear drops. If left untreated, a patient may lapse into a coma or even die, so urgent medical attention is required for patients in DKA and includes administering insulin and fluids, sometimes by IV injection. DKA occurs more often in type 1 DM patients. The other conditions are all chronic complications of diabetes caused by long-term hyperglycaemia which damages blood vessels. The chronic complications of DM cannot be reversed but need to be carefully managed as part of the patient's care.

15 **Which of the following is not a symptom of hypothyroidism?**

a) fatigue   b) unexplained weight gain   *c) diarrhoea*
d) sensitivity to cold

Constipation is a symptom of hypothyroidism due to the suppression of metabolic activity which slows down the motility in the gastrointestinal (GI) tract. Diarrhoea occurs when motility in the GI tract is too fast. Other symptoms of hypothyroidism include forgetfulness, numbness or tingling, muscle cramps, joint stiffness, tremors/poor coordination, dry skin, anaemia, fertility problems and high cholesterol.

FILL IN THE BLANKS

16 **Insulin is the main hormone that regulates cellular uptake of *glucose* from the blood.**

Insulin deficiency or the insensitivity of cell receptors to take up insulin, is characteristic of all forms of DM. Much of the dietary carbohydrate consumed is converted to glucose within a few hours. Insulin is released into the blood by beta cells located in the pancreatic islets of the pancreas, in response to an increasing blood glucose concentration after eating.

Higher insulin levels stimulate some anabolic (building up) processes such as cell growth and replication, protein synthesis and fat storage. If the amount of available insulin is insufficient, if cells are unresponsive to the effects of insulin (insulin resistance or insensitivity), or if the insulin is defective, then glucose will not be absorbed properly by the cells that require it for energy, nor will it be stored appropriately (as glycogen) in the liver and muscles. The overall effect is sustained high levels of blood glucose (hyperglycaemia), poor protein synthesis and other metabolic disorders, such as diabetic ketoacidosis (DKA) (see Answer 14).

17 **A patient with *Addison's* disease would exhibit symptoms including weight loss, dehydration and a craving for salty food.**

Other symptoms of this disease include fatigue, GI disturbances, muscle weakness, faintness, anxiety and (in pre-menopausal females) amenorrhoea. Patients can be treated with hydrocortisone and aldosterone and may expect to live a normal lifespan.

18 **A complication of *Cushing's* disease is associated hypertension which can lead to ischaemic heart disease.**

This is quite common in Cushing's disease and can ultimately lead to heart failure. Other complications include osteoporosis caused by increased calcium resorption from bones; peptic ulcers due to increased gastric secretions and impaired glucose tolerance caused by insulin resistance.

19 **Radioactive iodine therapy is the primary treatment for *hyperthyroidism*.**

Patients are administered radioactive iodine (^{131}I) which the thyroid gland absorbs in the same manner as regular iodine. The radioactivity destroys some of the cells in the thyroid gland that produce thyroxine (T_4) which reduces the thyroid hormone levels and so normalizes the size and function of the thyroid gland. In most patients the hypermetabolic symptoms disappear within four to eight weeks although some patients require a second treatment. This treatment is contraindicated during pregnancy. Surgery is recommended for patients who have had repeated relapse after drug therapy or who are allergic to ^{131}I.

20 **Thyroid hormone replacement is used in the treatment of *hypothyroidism*.**

Patients are treated with a synthetic thyroid hormone (levothyroxine). Treatment is usually introduced slowly to avoid adverse cardiac effects – especially in older patients. In under-developed countries, the incidence of hypothyroidism has decreased due to supplementing the diet with iodine, usually in the form of iodized table salt.

7 The cardiovascular system

INTRODUCTION

The heart and blood provide all the organs and tissues with nutrients and oxygen and remove waste. Diseases and disorders of the cardiovascular system may affect the heart, the blood and/or blood vessels and may be primary disorders of the system such as myocardial infarction (MI) or cerebrovascular accident (CVA) or secondary disorders caused by a condition arising in another organ system (for example, septicaemia arising as a complication of cellulitis). Disorders of the cardiovascular system affect many people during their lifetime.

Many of the signs and symptoms of cardiovascular system disorders can be general and vague at first. Often when specific symptoms arise and the patient presents for treatment, the damage to the heart and vessels of the circulatory system is irreversible. Acute cardiovascular disorders (MI or CVA) are considered medical emergencies because they can be life-threatening if not accurately diagnosed and treated rapidly.

Many public health campaigns now focus on raising awareness of disorders of this system, to help people reduce their risk of developing cardiovascular disease. In many instances, awareness and simple lifestyle adjustments may reduce risks and significantly improve life expectancy.

Nurses should appreciate that chronic or acute disruption or damage to the organs or vessels of the cardiovascular system can have serious and life-threatening consequences.

Useful resources

Nurses! Test Yourself in Anatomy and Physiology

Chapter 7

Ross and Wilson's Anatomy and Physiology in Health and Illness (11th edition)

Chapters 4 and 5

TRUE OR FALSE?

Are the following statements true or false?

1 Heart failure occurs as a result of impaired atrial function due to abnormality of the myocardial muscle.

2 When the atria distend in heart failure, there is a reflexive decrease in heart rate.

3 If the heart valves become damaged, abnormal murmurs can be heard.

4 All veins have corresponding arteries that run alongside each other.

5 Myocardial infarction (heart attack) is an acute coronary syndrome.

6 Hypertension is a decrease in blood pressure.

7 Cardiovascular disease describes disorders of the heart and its surrounding blood vessels.

8 Stable angina is classified as an acute coronary syndrome.

9 An aneurysm is an abnormal narrowing of an arterial wall.

10 Aneurysms are often asymptomatic.

11 The normal range for blood pH is 7.35–7.45.

12 Hypertension is a symptom of shock.

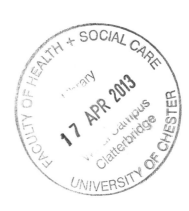

FACULTY OF HEALTH + SOCIAL CARE
Library
17 APR 2013
Campus
Clatterbridge
UNIVERSITY OF CHESTER

MULTIPLE CHOICE

Identify one correct answer for each of the following.

13 Which of the following is not a predisposing risk factor for myocardial infarction?

a) diabetes mellitus

b) elevated serum lipid levels

c) hypertension

d) cerebrovascular accident

14 Susceptibility to complications from myocardial infarction increases with:

a) age

b) body weight

c) serum lipid levels

d) hypertension

15 Coronary artery disease occurs when:

a) the body's glucose supply exceeds demand

b) the body's water demand exceeds supply

c) the body's oxygen demand exceeds supply

d) the body's oxygen supply exceeds demand

16 The main symptom of coronary artery disease is:

a) angina

b) breathlessness

c) cerebrovascular accident

d) headache

17 Which of these drug classes are used to prevent aneurysm rupture?

a) ACE-inhibitors

b) aspirin

c) beta-adrenoceptor blockers

d) non-steroidal anti-inflammatory drugs

18 How long does it take for cardiac troponins T and I to become elevated after a myocardial infarction?

a) within 30 seconds

b) within 10 minutes

c) within 4–6 hours

d) within 1–2 weeks

19 Which of these tests would identify the cause and severity of heart failure?

a) electrocardiogram

b) echocardiogram

c) cardiac enzymes

d) X-ray

20 Heart failure can usually be treated quickly with which type of drug?

a) beta-adrenoceptor blockers

b) diuretics

c) antiplatelet medications

d) anticoagulants

21 The immediate treatment for shock is:

a) give the patient a drink to calm him/her down

b) administer oxygen

c) identify the cause of the shock before administering treatment

d) lie the patient down with feet above the head

22 Which of the following is not a form of circulatory shock?

a) septic shock

b) cardiogenic shock

c) psychological shock

d) obstructive shock

23 Anaemia is caused by a deficiency of which essential element?

a) iron

b) oxygen

c) nitrogen

d) carbon

FILL IN THE BLANKS

Fill in the blanks in each statement using the options in this box.
Not all of them are required, so choose carefully!

---

myeloid	hypertension
MRI	irreversible
atherosclerosis	arteriosclerosis
pulmonary embolism	lymphoid
pacemaker	cardiac marker
electrocardiogram (ECG)	CVA
lymphocytic	

---

24 _____ does not produce any signs or symptoms until vascular damage has occurred in the heart, brain or kidneys.

25 The formation of atheroma on the inner walls of coronary arteries is called _____.

26 An artificial _____ may be fitted to stabilize arrhythmias following a myocardial infarction.

27 An _____ is the main tool used to diagnose angina or myocardial infarction.

28 A _____ _____ may develop as a complication of deep vein thrombosis.

29 _____ _____ enzymes are proteins used to diagnose myocardial infarction.

30 Leukaemia can be classified as acute or chronic and _____ or _____.

31 Chronic _____ leukaemia is the slowest and most benign form of leukaemia.

32 The _____ phase of shock cannot be corrected, even with medical intervention.

ANSWERS

TRUE OR FALSE?

1 **Heart failure occurs as a result of impaired atrial function due to abnormality of the myocardial muscle.**

Heart failure can occur when ventricular function (usually the left ventricle) is impaired due to cardiac muscle abnormalities. This abnormal muscle prevents the heart from pumping sufficient blood around the body to sustain oxygen and nutrient requirements of the tissues. The main symptom of heart failure is extreme tiredness due to the lack of oxygen getting to muscles and tissues. Other symptoms depend on the side of the heart affected. A left-sided failure will cause dyspnoea (breathlessness) while a right-sided failure can cause oedema in the ankles and legs due to accumulation of excess fluid. Fluid can also accumulate in the liver and stomach. Symptoms associated with failure on either (or both) sides of the heart include dizziness, loss of appetite, nausea and constipation.

2 **When the atria distend in heart failure, there is a reflexive decrease in heart rate.**

When the atria distend, there is a reflexive increase in the heart rate to pump the extra blood returning to the heart in venous return. Atrial distension can occur in heart failure or due to over-transfusion. When there is a sudden reduction in the pressure in the atria, the heartbeat slows. This is called the Bainbridge Reflex and is the cause of the significant bradycardia sometimes seen during spinal anaesthesia. It is best treated by elevating the legs to increase the venous return.

3 **If the heart valves become damaged, abnormal murmurs can be heard.**

The heart valves can be damaged through injury, disease (such as endocarditis or rheumatic fever) although damage is more commonly due to congenital abnormalities. Additional murmurs can be heard as the blood flows forwards through narrowed valves or leaks backwards through incompetent valves. Symptoms associated with aortic valve damage may not present until the damage is quite advanced. They include angina (because the heart is working harder to pump blood away) and dyspnoea, dizziness and fainting (all associated with the obstruction of blood flow from the heart). Abnormal murmurs can usually be detected with a stethoscope and require referral for further investigation.

4 | **All veins have corresponding arteries that run alongside each other.**

Deep veins have corresponding arteries that are usually located alongside each other; more superficial veins do not have corresponding arteries. At any given time, the majority of blood in the body is being transported through deep veins. Although most veins take blood back to the heart, there is an exception – the hepatic portal vein. Damage to this vein can be dangerous. Blood clotting in the hepatic portal vein can cause portal hypertension which results in a decrease of blood flow to the liver.

5 | **Myocardial infarction (heart attack) is an acute coronary syndrome.**

Acute coronary syndrome (ACS) is a term used to describe a range of thrombotic coronary artery diseases that cause acute ischaemia of the myocardial muscle tissue, namely unstable angina, ST-elevation MI (STEMI) and non-ST elevation MI (non-STEMI). All of these conditions are described as ACS because they reduce or impede blood flow through one of the coronary arteries causing ischaemia, injury and necrosis (infarction) to the tissue around the heart (see Figure 7.1). STEMI is the most serious ACS event because of the prolonged interruption of blood supply to the heart tissue, usually because the artery is completely occluded (blocked) (see Figure 7.2). A non-STEMI is less severe because the artery is only partly blocked, meaning blood supply is reduced but

Figure 7.1 Myocardial infarction

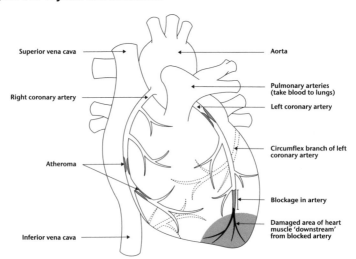

Figure 7.2 Section of an occluded coronary artery causing an MI

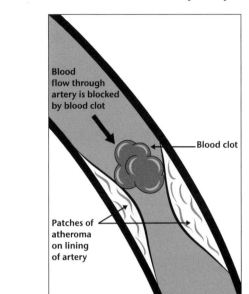

not completely impeded, therefore only part of the heart muscle being supplied by the affected artery is threatened. The different types of MI are diagnosed based on ECG observations (see Figure 7.3). Signs and symptoms of ACS are similar and are usually diagnosed from a detailed patient (and family) history, physical examination, electrocardiogram (ECG) and serum cardiac marker (enzyme) studies. ACS is a medical emergency and requires immediate hospital admission.

6 | Hypertension is a decrease in blood pressure.

Hypertension is an intermittent or sustained elevation of resting systolic and/or diastolic blood pressure (BP). It is caused by increases in cardiac output and/or peripheral resistance, making the heart work more. Resting systolic BP of greater than 140 mmHg is said to be high while a resting diastolic BP of greater than 90 mmHg is considered high. Therefore, a BP of 140/90 mmHg is said to be elevated. A BP of 120/100 mmHg is indicative of an elevated diastolic BP (since systolic value is still within normal range) while a BP of 160/60 mmHg is just high systolic pressure but normal diastolic range. Patients who have a sustained high BP are usually prescribed medication to help lower it. Hypertension is a risk factor for cardiovascular disease and kidney damage because sustained elevated blood pressure puts strain on the arteries, the heart and the delicate kidney vessels.

7 | **Cardiovascular disease describes disorders of the heart and its surrounding blood vessels.**

Cardiovascular diseases are diseases of the heart or blood vessels (vasculature). However, the term 'cardiovascular disease' is often used to describe diseases of the heart or blood vessels that are caused by atheroma (also known as atherosclerosis or hardening of the arteries). Patches of atheroma are small fatty lumps (or plaques) that develop on the inner, endothelial lining of arteries. Cardiovascular diseases that can be caused by atheroma include angina, MI, CVA and peripheral vascular disease.

8 | **Stable angina is classified as an acute coronary syndrome.**

Stable angina is not a symptom of acute coronary syndrome because it is not life-threatening. However, it is an important warning sign of an increased risk of more serious conditions, such as MI or CVA.

Unstable angina is a symptom of acute coronary syndrome because symptoms develop rapidly, can persist even at rest, and can last up to 30 minutes. It is much more likely to develop into an MI than stable angina. It can sometimes be relieved by nitrates (such as glyceryl trinitrate (GTN)) which relax and dilate the blood vessels, increasing the blood supply to the heart. However, sometimes angina can be resistant to this treatment. Upon admission to hospital, patients are usually administered anticoagulant medication (such as heparin) to prevent MI. Other drugs can be used to control and reduce risk of acute coronary disease, including beta-adrenoceptor blockers (beta-blockers) or angiotensin-converting enzyme (ACE) inhibitors as well as statins to control serum cholesterol levels.

9 | **An aneurysm is an abnormal narrowing of an arterial wall.**

An aneurysm is abnormal dilation (stretching or widening) of an arterial wall. Aneurysms can occur in the brain (cerebral or intracranial aneurysm) or aorta (known as abdominal aortic aneurysm). In an abdominal aortic aneurysm, this dilation occurs in the aorta between the renal arteries and the iliac branches. Aneurysms are more common in males than females. They usually develop due to a muscular weakness in the artery wall that allows the vessel to stretch outward. Blood pressure (especially high BP) can weaken the vessel wall and increase the size of the aneurysm. Narrowing of arterial walls is caused by accumulation of atherosclerotic plaques (atheroma) on the inner layer (intima) of the walls of the coronary arteries. When a blood clot attaches to atheroma, blood supply to cardiac tissue can be reduced and this may result in angina or an MI (see Figures 7.1 and 7.2).

10 | **Aneurysms are often asymptomatic.**

Many aneurysms do not produce symptoms and are only detected on an X-ray or CT scan during routine physical examination or if there is a family history. In many cases, the exact cause of an aneurysm is unclear, although risk factors include smoking, hypertension and a family history of aneurysms.

11　**The normal range for blood pH is 7.35–7.45.**

The normal pH range of circulating blood is maintained by buffer systems, the lungs and the kidneys. When these systems are functioning normally together, they neutralize and eliminate acids as quickly as they are formed.

12　**Hypertension is a symptom of shock.**

Shock is an acute condition caused when the circulatory system fails, depriving the tissues of oxygen and nutrients and indicated by hypotension (low blood pressure). This is circulatory (or physiological) shock and should not be confused with emotional shock. Circulatory shock can be severe and potentially life-threatening. It can be caused by: (1) a fall in cardiac output after a haemorrhage or other fluid loss; (2) damage to the heart after an MI; (3) external pressure on the heart; or (4) extensive peripheral vasodilation such as in an anaphylactic hypersensitivity reaction. Other symptoms of shock include pale or clammy skin, confusion/disorientation, rapid shallow breathing, rapid weak pulse, nausea or vomiting, and thirst. Respiratory acidosis may develop as a complication due to the drop in blood pH (see Chapter 8, Answer 8).

 MULTIPLE CHOICE

Correct answers identified in bold italics

13　**Which of the following is not a predisposing risk factor for myocardial infarction?**

a) diabetes mellitus　b) elevated serum lipid levels　c) hypertension
d) cerebrovascular accident (CVA)

A history of CVA is not associated with increased risk of MI. MI is caused by an occlusion (blockage) of a coronary artery, the occlusion can be due to a number of factors such as atherosclerosis, thrombosis, or platelet aggregation (clumping). Many of the predisposing factors for MI or ACS are lifestyle-related and include sedentary lifestyle, high salt diet, obesity, smoking, stress, use of recreational drugs. Non-lifestyle factors include increasing age and a family history of coronary artery disease (CAD).

14　**Susceptibility to complications from myocardial infarction increases with:**

a) age　b) body weight　c) serum lipid levels　d) hypertension

Risk of complications and death associated with MI increases with patient's age. Complications include arrhythmias, cardiogenic shock, or heart failure, causing pulmonary oedema, or rupture of chamber walls or valves.

15 **Coronary artery disease occurs when:**

a) the body's glucose supply exceeds demand
b) the body's water demand exceeds supply
c) the body's oxygen demand exceeds supply
d) the body's oxygen supply exceeds demand

Coronary artery disease (CAD) reduces the supply of oxygen and nutrients to myocardial tissues due to poor coronary blood flow. The most common cause of CAD is atherosclerosis, when fatty, fibrous plaques (atheroma) accumulate. This narrows the inner lining of the walls of arteries supplying the heart, thus reducing the volume of blood that can flow through the vessels. Many of the risk factors associated with CAD are modifiable, so patients can help to reduce their risks of developing CAD or the associated MI, by making minor lifestyle adjustments, such as eating a diet low in saturated fat and taking regular moderate exercise.

16 **The main symptom of coronary artery disease is:**

a) angina   b) breathlessness   c) cerebrovascular accident
d) headache

Angina is a classic sign of coronary artery disease. Patients may report a crushing, squeezing or burning pain in the left side of the chest that radiates down the left arm and sometimes upwards into the neck and jaw – the same type of pain experienced in an MI. The pain is often accompanied by nausea, vomiting, fainting or sweating, although not all patients, especially females, report the classic pain symptoms of angina or MI. Symptoms usually occur after physical exertion or high emotions but can develop during rest or even sleep.

17 **Which of these drug classes are used to prevent aneurysm rupture?**

a) ACE-inhibitors   b) aspirin   *c) beta-adrenoceptor blockers*
d) non-steroidal anti-inflammatory drugs

Beta-adrenoceptor blockers (beta-blockers) are usually prescribed to decrease the extension of an aneurysm and prevent rupture but surgery may be required if the aneurysm is quite large or at risk of rupture. An alternative to surgical resection (removal) of the aneurysm is a stent graft, where the damaged section of the blood vessel is replaced with a piece of supportive tubing. Symptoms of a ruptured aneurysm include sweating, weakness and tachycardia. A ruptured aortic aneurysm will also be accompanied by severe abdominal pain. If left untreated, a ruptured aneurysm will result in death, although before shock sets in, patients may remain quite stable for a number of hours before death. A ruptured aortic aneurysm will be fatal in 65–85 per cent of patients.

18 **How long does it take for cardiac troponins T and I to become elevated after a myocardial infarction?**

a) within 30 seconds   b) within 10 minutes   *c) within 4–6 hours*
d) within 1–2 weeks

The cardiac troponins (cTn) T and I are released within 4–6 hours of an MI and peak between 24 and 48 hours. They remain elevated above baseline levels for up to two weeks after the attack and are almost completely specific to myocardial tissue. Therefore they are the preferred markers for assessing myocardial damage over other cardiac enzymes such as creatine kinase (CK), aspartate aminotransferase (AST) or lactate dehydrogenase (LAD), which all have much lower specificity for cardiac muscle compared to troponins T and I. Troponin is a contractile protein not normally found in serum. It is only released when myocardial necrosis occurs. Cardiac troponins T and I are highly sensitive and specific to myocardial tissue damage. Troponins T and I are of equal clinical value; when elevated troponins are detected along with chest pain, it is considered a strong predictor of MI in the near future. The risk of death from an ACS is directly related to troponin levels, patients with no detectable troponins have a positive short-term prognosis.

19 **Which of these tests would identify the cause and severity of heart failure?**

a) electrocardiogram   *b) echocardiogram*   c) cardiac enzymes
d) X-ray

An echocardiogram is an ultrasound scan that evaluates the pumping action of the heart. It will help identify the underlying cause, type and severity of heart failure. A chest X-ray will determine if the heart is enlarged and if there is fluid in the lungs while an ECG records the electrical activity and rhythms of the heart. A number of cardiac enzymes are released by the myocardial cells following damage due to an MI.

20 **Heart failure can usually be treated quickly with which type of drug?**

a) beta-adrenoceptor blockers   *b) diuretics*
c) antiplatelet medications   d) anticoagulants

The immediate treatment of heart failure usually consists of a combination of diuretics and vasodilators. Diuretics such as furosemide are administered to reduce blood volume and the resulting congestion in the circulatory system. Vasodilators (namely ACE-inhibitors) allow the arteries to relax and dilate and increase cardiac output, making it easier for the heart to pump blood around the body. Anticoagulants, such as warfarin, and antiplatelet treatment, such as aspirin, thin the blood and therefore help prevent stroke. These are recommended for the management of chronic heart failure but should not be used in combination because their combined effects may cause haemorrhage. Beta-adrenoceptor blockers are not commonly used to treat heart failure in an emergency but can be used in long-term management of chronic heart failure.

21 | **The immediate treatment for shock is:**

a) give the patient a drink to calm him/her down
b) administer oxygen
c) identify the cause of the shock before administering treatment
d) lie the patient down with feet above the head

Ideally the feet should be elevated above the head, which will help raise the blood pressure and preserve blood flow to the brain. If the brain is starved of oxygen, the tissue will begin to die and damage will be irreversible. Treatment should also aim to stop any bleeding by applying direct pressure over the wound or a tourniquet on extreme limb injuries. A patient suffering from suspected shock should never be given anything to eat or drink because of the risk of vomiting. If the patient is experiencing anaphylactic shock and is conscious but having trouble breathing, it is best to sit them upright.

22 | **Which of the following is not a form of circulatory shock?**

a) septic shock   b) cardiogenic shock   *c) psychological shock*
d) obstructive shock

Psychological (emotional) shock should not be confused with circulatory (or physiological) shock. Psychological shock can occur after a physically or emotionally traumatic experience and affects the state of mind. It can produce symptoms such as palpitations and faintness, but it does not usually lead to serious physical collapse. Septic shock, cardiogenic shock and obstructive shock are forms of circulatory shock which are not caused by low blood volume but are still life-threatening. Septic shock is caused by bacteria releasing massive amounts of toxins during a systemic infection, causing peripheral vasodilation and a dangerous drop in blood pressure. Symptoms are similar to other circulatory shocks but patients may exhibit a fever due to the infection. Cardiogenic shock occurs when the heart is unable to maintain a normal cardiac output – often caused by a failure in the left ventricle after MI. Thrombolytic (clot-busting) drugs can restore coronary circulation and relieve symptoms. Other causes of cardiogenic shock include arrhythmias, valve disorders and advanced coronary heart disease. Obstructive shock occurs when ventricular output is reduced when fluid or tissue restricts the beating of the heart. It is often caused by fluid build up in the pericardial cavity (cardiac tamponade).

23 | **Anaemia is caused by a deficiency of which essential element?**

a) iron   b) oxygen   c) nitrogen   d) carbon

If there is a lack of iron in the diet, a patient can develop anaemia which means the production of haemoglobin is reduced, which affects the ability of the red blood cells to carry and distribute oxygen around the body. Normal haemoglobin levels are in the range of 130–180 g/L in males and between 120 and 160 g/L in females. Values in children vary with age. Other causes of anaemia include pregnancy, excess blood loss (perhaps due to bleeding ulcer or injury) or conditions that result in poor iron absorption from food. Symptoms usually include fatigue, poor concentration, tachycardia and paleness (especially of conjunctivae and nail beds). Treatment usually involves an oral iron supplement (sometimes in combination with ascorbic acid (vitamin C) which enhances iron absorption) and dietary advice to increase iron consumption.

FILL IN THE BLANKS

24 *Hypertension* **does not produce any signs or symptoms until vascular damage has occurred in the heart, brain or kidneys.**

Hypertension is asymptomatic (has no symptoms) when it first begins but if left untreated, sustained hypertension damages the lining of blood vessels and can produce major complications that can be fatal. Symptoms that may develop in brain include transient ischaemic attack (TIA) or stroke, or blindness can develop due to damage to the blood vessels of the retina. Hypertension can cause an MI while prolonged protein in urine (proteinuria) and oedema can result in renal failure.

25 **The formation of atheroma on the inner walls of coronary arteries is called** *atherosclerosis.*

Atherosclerosis is a form of arteriosclerosis characterized by the deposition of atheroma containing cholesterol and lipids on the innermost membrane (tunica intima) of the walls of large and medium-sized arteries. Individuals with atherosclerosis have a higher risk of coronary artery disease and stroke. Smoking, hypertension, diabetes mellitus, and elevated levels of saturated fat in the blood contribute to the development of atherosclerosis. Arteriosclerosis describes the thickening, hardening, and loss of elasticity of the arterial walls that results in impaired blood circulation, it is associated with increasing age as well as hypertension, diabetes mellitus and poor diet.

26 **An artificial** *pacemaker* **may be fitted to stabilize arrhythmias following a myocardial infarction.**

Arrhythmias are the most common problem immediately after an MI and stabilizing these is one of the three goals of MI treatment. The others are to relieve chest pain and reduce the workload of the heart. A pacemaker may be fitted temporarily to stabilize heartbeat and treat life-threatening bradycardia. To relieve chest pain, a patient would usually be treated with IV morphine and beta-blockers to reduce the workload of the heart. In addition, patients may be prescribed statins if their serum cholesterol levels are elevated.

27 **An** *electrocardiogram (ECG)* **is the main tool used to diagnose angina or myocardial infarction.**

An ECG can be used to diagnose angina and will show ischaemia in the form of an inverted T-wave, ST-segment depression and possibly arrhythmias (Figure 7.3).

Figure 7.3 ECG patterns in MI

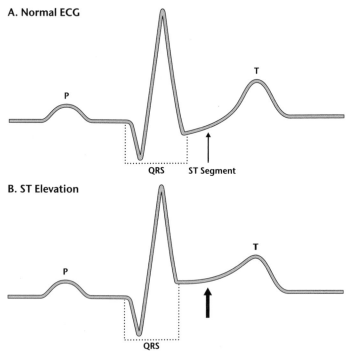

A. Normal ECG

P

QRS ST Segment

T

B. ST Elevation

P

QRS

T

ST Elevation: Observed when acute heart damage has occurred due to MI – would indicate a STEMI.

C. ST Depression

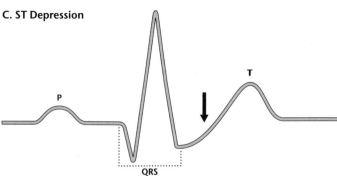

P

QRS

T

ST Depression: Indicates ischaemia has occurred but is not a sign of infarction. Patient may experience pain. T wave may also be flattened or inverted. Treatment with digoxin can produce ST depression and inverted T wave.

This pattern is also caused by biochemical conditions such as hypokalaemia, hypocalcaemia or hypomagnesaemia and may be observed in cases of hypothermia.

28 | A *pulmonary embolism* may develop as a complication of deep vein thrombosis.

Deep vein thrombosis (DVT) is a blood clot in one of the deep veins in the body, it usually occurs in a deep leg vein that runs through the muscles of the calf and thigh. It can cause pain and swelling in the leg. Complications such as pulmonary embolism may arise when a piece of blood clot breaks off, travels in the bloodstream and blocks one of the blood vessels in the lungs. DVT and pulmonary embolism together are known as venous thromboembolism (VTE). Anyone can develop DVT although there are some risk factors such as a family history of thrombosis, pregnancy, medical conditions (cancer or heart failure), inactivity (for example, after an operation) and obesity. Sometimes DVT may be asymptomatic, although symptoms include pain, swelling and a heavy ache in the leg, a warm feeling around the affected area and redness on the skin around the area. Symptoms of a pulmonary embolism are more serious and include: breathlessness, which may come on gradually or suddenly, chest pain, which may be worse when inhaling, or sudden collapse. If symptoms of DVT or pulmonary embolism develop, urgent medical attention should be sought as these conditions may be life-threatening. DVT is usually treated with anticoagulants such as warfarin or heparin. Heparin may be used in emergencies to thin the blood and is suitable for use during pregnancy (whereas warfarin is not). Patients will also be advised to elevate their leg and wear compression stockings to relieve pressure on the leg veins and prevent fluid accumulation in the calf.

29 | *Cardiac marker* enzymes are proteins used to diagnose myocardial infarction.

An MI diagnosis requires two out of three components, namely history, ECG and cardiac marker enzymes. When damage to the heart occurs, levels of cardiac markers rise over time, which is why blood tests are taken over a 24-hour period. The specific enzymes that are measured to diagnose MI are creatinine kinase (CK) and cardiac troponins. Troponins T and I are specific to myocardial injury, although these enzyme levels are not elevated immediately following an MI. If patients present with chest pain, they are generally treated on the assumption that an MI has occurred and then evaluated over time for a more precise diagnosis.

30 | Leukaemia can be classified as acute or chronic and *lymphoid* or *myeloid*.

Leukaemia describes a group of malignant disorders of the white blood cells (WBCs). In acute leukaemia, immature WBCs accumulate in the body and disrupt the function of organs and tissues. In chronic leukaemias cells are slightly abnormal and therefore do not function properly. Lymphoid refers to lymphocytes (type of white blood cell) that arise from lymphoid stem cells while the remaining WBCs arise from myeloid stem cells. Risks associated with acute leukaemias are increased by smoking, exposure to radiation and treatment for a previous cancer diagnosis. Symptoms for all leukaemias are vague and include fatigue, weight loss, frequent infections and anaemia. If untreated, acute leukaemias progress rapidly and aggressively. They can be fatal and prognosis varies with treatment and type of disease. Acute lymphocytic leukaemia (ALL) accounts for about 80 per cent of childhood leukaemias while acute myeloid leukaemia (AML) is one of the most common leukaemias in adults.

31 **Chronic *lymphocytic* leukaemia is the slowest and most benign form of leukaemia.**

Chronic lymphocytic leukaemia (CLL) is a progressive disease which causes a proliferation and accumulation of malfunctioning, immune-deficient lymphocytes. Risk increases with age and hereditary factors are thought to be involved in CLL which is more common in males. Chronic myeloid leukaemia (CML) is caused by excessive development of granulocytes in the bone marrow, which circulate in the blood and infiltrate the liver and spleen. CML risk increases with age and exposure to radiation and carcinogenic chemicals (such as benzene). Some signs and symptoms for both types of chronic leukaemia are similar to acute leukaemias and include fatigue, weight loss and frequent infections. For chronic leukaemias, there may also be swelling of lymph glands, liver and enlargement of the spleen (splenomegaly). Tests for CLL usually include lymph node biopsy which distinguishes benign and malignant tumours, while routine blood tests will usually identify an increasing lymphocyte count along with low haemoglobin levels. Tests for CML would include bone marrow biopsy to check for bone marrow infiltration along with WBC count. CT scans would identify affected organs and tissues.

32 **The *irreversible* phase of shock cannot be corrected, even with medical intervention.**

In the absence of treatment, circulatory shock will progress into irreversible (or refractory) shock when the heart, liver, kidneys and central nervous system rapidly begin to deteriorate and eventually fail. This cannot be reversed, even with medical intervention. It happens when the conditions in the tissues become so abnormal that the arterioles and capillaries are unable to contract and so widespread peripheral vasodilation occurs which causes a fatal drop in blood pressure. This event is called circulatory collapse. Blood flow through the capillaries stops and the tissues quickly begin to die by necrosis, effects that spread rapidly throughout the body.

8 The respiratory system

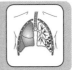

INTRODUCTION

The respiratory system consists of the lungs, respiratory airways and the associated blood vessels.

Disease or trauma to the respiratory system can affect the lungs, respiratory airways, breathing mechanics or the nervous and endocrine control of ventilation. Respiratory disorders can often be classified as acute or chronic. Chronic disorders often arise as a complication in patients who are already immunocompromised. Symptoms of many respiratory disorders are similar, such as shortness of breath, cough, wheezing.

Peak expiratory flow rate, chest X-ray, bronchoscopy and tissue specimens are common diagnostic tools used in respiratory investigations.

Treatment of many chronic respiratory disorders aims to alleviate symptoms while preventing the patient's condition from further deteriorating. In acute conditions, the priority is to accurately diagnose the disease or illness and commence appropriate treatment quickly.

Nurses are often responsible for the ventilation of patients in a number of treatment settings such as high dependency units (HDUs) or intensive care units (ICUs), so it is important to be familiar with the disorders and treatment of these respiratory conditions.

Useful resources

Nurses! Test Yourself in Anatomy and Physiology

Chapter 8

Ross and Wilson's Anatomy and Physiology in Health and Illness (11th edition)

Chapter 10

TRUE OR FALSE?

Are the following statements true or false?

1 Asthma is a chronic disorder of the alveoli.

2 The best advice for patients living with asthma is to try to prevent an attack.

3 Pneumonia is an acute infection of the bronchi.

4 Fungal infection of the lungs is the most common cause of pneumonia.

5 Chronic respiratory disease can increase the risk of developing pneumonia.

6 Small-cell lung cancer is more common than non-small-cell lung cancer.

7 Spontaneous and traumatic pneumothorax present with different signs and symptoms.

8 Respiratory acidosis is a potential complication of chronic obstructive pulmonary disorders.

MULTIPLE CHOICE

Identify one correct answer for each of the following.

9 Asthma can be classified as which type of respiratory condition?

    a) bronchitis

    b) chronic obstructive pulmonary disorder (COPD)

    c) pneumonia

    d) respiratory failure

10 What is the main risk factor for chronic obstructive pulmonary disorder?

    a) smoking

    b) environmental exposure to toxins

    c) family history

    d) frequent respiratory infections

11 Which of the following is not a symptom of asthma?

    a) cough

    b) wheezing

    c) chest tightening

    d) chest infection

12 Pneumonia can be classified in how many ways?

    a) 1

    b) 2

    c) 3

    d) 4

13 Which type of pneumonia will respond best to treatment with antibiotics?

a) viral

b) bacterial

c) fungal

d) protozoal

14 Which of the following would identify the type of pneumonia infection?

a) sputum culture

b) chest X-ray

c) pulse oximetry

d) arterial blood gas analysis

15 Which type of lung cancer has the most rapid growth and metastasis rate?

a) adenocarcinoma

b) large-cell

c) small-cell

d) squamous cell

FILL IN THE BLANKS

Fill in the blanks in each statement using the options in this box.
Not all of them are required, so choose carefully!

bacterial	pneumothorax
peak expiratory	bronchoscopy
salmeterol	viral
effusion	salbutamol
ECG	spirometery

16 The most common diagnostic test for asthma is the _____ _____ flow rate test.

17 _____ is a short-acting beta$_2$ agonist, used to treat asthma symptoms.

18 *Streptococcus pneumoniae* is the most common cause of _____ pneumonia.

19 _____ is a common diagnostic tool used in all types of lung cancers.

20 _____ is an accumulation of air in the pleural cavity leading to partial or complete lung collapse.

MATCH THE TERMS

Match each respiratory condition with the appropriate classification:

A. infection

B. degenerative

C. congenital

| 21 | Acute bronchitis _____ |

| 22 | Chronic bronchitis _____ |

| 23 | Cystic fibrosis _____ |

| 24 | Emphysema _____ |

ANSWERS

TRUE OR FALSE?

1 **Asthma is a chronic disorder of the alveoli.**

Asthma is a chronic disorder of the bronchi. During an acute episode, airflow in and out of the lungs is impaired due to narrowing and obstruction of the airways caused by bronchospasm (narrowing of the bronchi when the smooth muscle contracts). Together with irritation, bronchospasm triggers increased mucus secretions and oedema of the mucosa.

2 **The best advice for patients living with asthma is to try to prevent an attack.**

Knowing and avoiding triggers is the best attitude with all COPD conditions. The main pharmacological (drug) treatment for the relief of asthma symptoms is the beta$_2$-adrenoceptor agonists (or beta$_2$ agonists) which act as bronchodilators by mimicking the action of adrenaline; they can be short-acting or longer-acting. Short-acting treatments, such as salbutamol, work within five minutes of administration to relieve symptoms by relaxing the airway muscles and decreasing the mucus secretion for 3–6 hours. Patients who have mild, intermittent asthma symptoms are advised to avoid triggers and would be prescribed beta$_2$ agonists to be taken when they experience symptoms. People who suffer from more frequent symptoms would be prescribed inhaled corticosteroids (steroids) to prevent symptoms, the dose and type of corticosteroid would be determined by the severity of symptoms. Patients would also be prescribed a beta$_2$ agonist to relieve symptoms when they occur.

3 **Pneumonia is an acute infection of the bronchi.**

Pneumonia is an acute infection of the alveoli that impairs gas exchange. It occurs when the protective processes fail to prevent inhaled or blood-borne microbes entering and colonizing the lungs. Prognosis is good for patients with normal lung function and an adequate immune system but bacterial pneumonia is the leading cause of death in debilitated patients.

4 **Fungal infection of the lungs is the most common cause of pneumonia.**

Bacteria are the most common cause of pneumonia. Fungal pneumonia is relatively uncommon but may occur in individuals who are immuno-suppressed or have immune system disorders such as HIV/AIDS. The pathophysiology of pneumonia caused by fungi is similar to that of bacterial pneumonia.

5 | Chronic respiratory disease can increase the risk of developing pneumonia.

There are a number of other predisposing factors that can increase the risk of developing bacterial and viral pneumonia such as chronic debilitating illness, lung cancer, cystic fibrosis, smoking or malnutrition. Premature babies are also at greater risk of developing pneumonia due to the under-developed state of their lungs at birth. Aspiration pneumonia is a risk for patients who are debilitated, unconscious or receiving food through a nasogastric tube.

6 | Small-cell lung cancer is more common than non-small-cell lung cancer.

Non-small-cell lung cancer (NSCLC) accounts for about 80 per cent of all lung cancers. There are three subtypes of NSCLC: adenocarcinoma, squamous cell and large-cell. Only 20 per cent of lung cancers are small-cell (SCLC) type; this is primarily found in smokers. Non-smokers rarely develop SCLC. The general prognosis for lung cancer is poor. Lung cancer is considered a preventable disease and arises from repeated damage to lung epithelial tissue caused by inhaling irritants or carcinogens such as tobacco smoke, air pollution, asbestos and radon gas.

7 | Spontaneous and traumatic pneumothorax present with different signs and symptoms.

Although the causes of each type are quite different, they exhibit similar symptoms, these include a sudden sharp chest pain, exacerbated by breathing and coughing, shortness of breath, cyanosis and respiratory distress. Tension pneumothorax is a dangerous complication that can develop when air is unable to escape from the thoracic cavity, causing pressure to increase around the heart and its major blood vessels. Tension pneumothorax causes severe symptoms such as hypotension, decreased cardiac output, tachycardia and cardiac arrest and should be treated as a medical emergency.

8 | Respiratory acidosis is a potential complication of chronic obstructive pulmonary disorders.

Respiratory acidosis can be caused by diseases or conditions that affect gas exchange in the lungs, such as emphysema, chronic bronchitis, asthma, or severe pneumonia. Blockage of the airways (due to swelling or by a foreign object) impairs gas exchange which can lead to an accumulation of acidic carbon dioxide in the blood. This can induce respiratory acidosis because the blood pH becomes more acidic (drops below pH 7.35). Respiratory acidosis can also be caused by an abnormal control of breathing from the respiratory control centre in the medulla oblongata of the brain (perhaps due to a head injury or stroke). The main symptom is slow, difficult breathing, which may be accompanied by headache, but drowsiness, restlessness, tremor and confusion may also occur. A rapid heart rate, changes in blood pressure and swelling of blood vessels in the eyes may be observed and the patient may appear cyanosed (blue/purple in colour) due to hypoxia (lack of oxygen). Respiratory acidosis is diagnosed from arterial blood gas (ABG) readings, indicating high carbon dioxide levels. The underlying condition should be treated but patients may be given oxygen therapy and bronchodilators to ease breathing. If untreated, severe cases of respiratory acidosis can lead to coma and death.

MULTIPLE CHOICE

Correct answers identified in bold italics

9 **Asthma can be classified as which type of respiratory condition?**

a) bronchitis　　*b) chronic obstructive pulmonary disorder (COPD)*
c) pneumonia　　d) respiratory failure

COPD is the classification for chronic, long-term, respiratory disorders that are characterized by obstruction of the airways. Chronic bronchitis and emphysema are also types of COPD. Pneumonia is an acute infection of the lungs that affects gas exchange. In respiratory failure, the lungs cannot obtain enough oxygen (or eliminate sufficient carbon dioxide) which results in the body tissues being starved of oxygen (tissue hypoxia) and being overcome by an accumulation of CO_2 (hypercapnia). COPD patients are at risk of acute respiratory failure if their arterial blood gas values deteriorate.

10 **What is the main risk factor for chronic obstructive pulmonary disorder?**

a) smoking　　b) environmental exposure to toxins　　c) family history
d) frequent respiratory infections

Smoking impairs the action and destroys the cilia of the epithelial cells that line the respiratory tract. It also damages the immune action of the macrophages. Together these trigger inflammation of the airways which increases mucus production, causing alveolar dysfunction and fibrosis (scarring) of the bronchioles. Exposure to environmental toxins such as asbestos, family history and recurring respiratory infections are also risk factors for COPD.

11 **Which of the following is not a symptom of asthma?**

a) cough　　b) wheezing　　c) chest tightening　　*d) chest infection*

Cough, wheezing, chest tightening and difficulty breathing are symptoms of asthma. Symptoms depend on the severity of the patient's asthma:

- The least severe form of the disease is mild and intermittent; these patients are symptom-free between attacks.

- An individual who experiences symptoms a few times a week is classified as having mild persistent asthma.

- Patients who experience symptoms daily and have normal or below normal air exchange have moderate, persistent asthma.

- Those with severe persistent asthma experience symptoms continually and have below normal air exchange. The physical activity of such patients is compromised by their severe symptoms. Chest infections (such as pneumonia) may develop as a complication of asthma. Patients with underlying respiratory conditions may require hospital treatment such as IV fluids, antibiotics and oxygen therapy if they develop complications.

12 Pneumonia can be classified in how many ways?

a) 1   b) 2   *c) 3*   d) 4

Pneumonia can be classified according to its infecting pathogen, affected location in the lungs, or whether it is primary, secondary or aspiration pneumonia. The infectious pathogen may be bacterial, viral, fungal or protozoal in nature. Bacteria and fungi are the most common pathogens. If pneumonia is classified as bronchopneumonia, there will be infected patches in both lungs, while lobar pneumonia involves part of or an entire lobe. Primary pneumonia results from inhaling an infectious pathogen. Secondary pneumonia can follow lung tissue damage from inhaling a noxious chemical or bacterial spread. Aspiration pneumonia is caused by inhaling foreign matter into the bronchi (such as food particles or vomitus (vomit particles)).

13 Which type of pneumonia will respond best to treatment with antibiotics?

a) viral   *b) bacterial*   c) fungal   d) protozoal

Antibiotic treatment will only be successful when treating a condition that is bacterial in origin. Sometimes patients with viral, fungal or protozoal pneumonias develop a secondary bacterial infection. In this situation, antibiotics may be prescribed to treat the secondary bacterial infection but will not treat the underlying pathogenic cause of the pneumonia.

14 Which of the following would identify the type of pneumonia infection?

a) sputum culture   b) chest X-ray   c) pulse oximetry
d) arterial blood gas analysis

Sputum culture and Gram's staining help differentiate the type of infection and therefore indicate the most effective drugs for treatment because antibiotics will be ineffective in treating a viral pneumonia. Chest X-ray can confirm diagnosis by identifying infiltrates but it does not always confirm pneumonia. Pulse oximetry may indicate reduced oxygen saturation levels. ABG levels vary with the severity of the pneumonia. Blood culture can indicate the specific bacteria if the disease is bacterial in nature. Bronchoscopy may be performed to collect culture material for diagnosis.

15 **Which type of lung cancer has the most rapid growth and metastasis rate?**

a) adenocarcinoma   b) large-cell   **c) *small-cell***   d) squamous cell

Small-cell lung cancer (SCLC) grows most rapidly and metastasizes very early, yet it responds very well to chemotherapy treatment. Unfortunately any response is relatively short due to the very rapid growth and potential for metastasis of SCLC. Large-cell lung cancer is also rapid growing and metastasis occurs quite early on in disease development (but not as rapidly as SCLC). Adenocarcinoma is the most common type of lung cancer. It is a moderate-growing lung cancer but with quite early metastasis. The slowest growing type of lung cancer is squamous cell tumours, these are also quite slow to metastasize.

FILL IN THE BLANKS

16 **The most common diagnostic test for asthma is the _peak expiratory_ flow rate test.**

The peak expiratory flow rate test (PEFR or peak flow) uses a peak flow meter to measure the speed at which air is exhaled from the lungs. A reading is taken and the patient is then treated with a beta$_2$ agonist that treats asthma by relaxing the bronchial muscles (bronchodilation) and reducing mucus secretion for a short period of time. A second reading is then taken. If the reading is much higher after taking the beta$_2$ agonist, then the diagnosis is confirmed. Patients with additional symptoms may be referred for a chest X-ray to exclude other lung conditions.

17 **_Salbutamol_ is a short-acting beta$_2$ agonist, used to treat asthma symptoms.**

Salbutamol is a short-acting beta$_2$ agonist which mimics the action of the natural hormone adrenaline by causing bronchodilation. Longer-acting beta$_2$ agonists are usually administered following treatment with a short-acting drug. They treat symptoms in the same way as short-acting drugs but take around 30 minutes to act and effects last up to 12 hours. Salmeterol is a long-acting beta$_2$ agonist. In addition to beta$_2$ agonist treatment, patients with moderate/persistent symptoms may be prescribed inhaled corticosteroids (hydrocortisone or methylprednisolone) which have anti-inflammatory effects as well as causing bronchodilation as part of the long-term control of asthma.

18 | *Streptococcus pneumoniae* **is the most common cause of** *bacterial* **pneumonia.**

These bacteria invade the lungs and settle in the alveoli where they cause an immune response that induces pneumonia symptoms namely, fever, chills, shortness of breath and fatigue (common in bacterial and fungal pneumonia). Complications arise when bacteria enter the blood from the infected lung, causing serious or even fatal illness such as septic shock.

19 | *Bronchoscopy* **is a common diagnostic tool used in all types of lung cancers.**

Bronchoscopy is used to identify the tumour site and often to retrieve tissue specimens for histological examination. Needle biopsy is often used to locate tumours in the peripheral regions of the lungs and to collect tissue for analysis. Chest X-ray is used to locate an advanced lesion while bone and CT scans are often performed to investigate for metastases.

20 | *Pneumothorax* **is an accumulation of air in the pleural cavity leading to partial or complete lung collapse.**

Pneumothorax can be classified as spontaneous or traumatic. It is usually diagnosed by chest X-ray. Spontaneous pneumothorax most often occurs in patients with chronic pulmonary disorders and in young men (and is often sports-related). Traumatic pneumothorax can have a number of causes such as crushing trauma to the chest (perhaps causing broken ribs), penetrating wound (stabbing, gunshot) and during surgical procedures. If venous return is impeded, a serious complication can develop known as tension pneumothorax (see Answer 7). A small pneumothorax usually clears without treatment over a few days as the body heals the leak and the air is gradually absorbed. For a larger pneumothorax the air must be removed to relieve symptoms either with a syringe and needle, or by inserting a chest drain (placing a drainage tube into the space to allow the air to escape) which may need to stay in place until the lung heals. With a tension pneumothorax, immediate medical treatment is required to relieve the life-threatening symptoms; the air is released by putting a large bore hollow needle directly into the chest.

MATCH THE TERMS

21 | Acute bronchitis   **A.** infection

- *Pathophysiology*: Bronchitis is an inflammation of the bronchi which causes an over-production of mucus causing frequent coughing.

- *Causes*: Acute bronchitis can be caused by a bacterial or viral infection but viral infections (usually the same viruses that cause colds and influenza) spread by coughing and sneezing are most common.

- *Risk factors*: Anyone can develop bronchitis but it can occur with a cold or influenza and is linked with exposure to damp environments.

- *Symptoms*: Productive cough (the cough expels mucus) is the main symptom but it may be accompanied by wheezing, tightness in the chest and other flu-like symptoms.

- *Diagnosis and treatment*: Many cases of acute bronchitis will clear on their own within a few weeks (described as self-limiting). A diagnosis is made by listening to the chest and considering the symptoms. Treatment is similar to that for a cold or mild influenza, namely rest and plenty of fluids (to thin out the mucus in the lungs and prevent dehydration). Paracetamol or ibuprofen can be prescribed for aches and pains. Patients are advised to consult a GP if they have an underlying heart or lung condition. An antibiotic will not normally be prescribed (because acute bronchitis is usually caused by viral infection) but if a patient is at risk of pneumonia, a prophylactic (preventative) antibiotic may be recommended.

- *Complications*: Repeated episodes of acute bronchitis can cause permanent damage to the airways resulting in chronic bronchitis.

22 Chronic bronchitis   **B. degenerative**

- *Pathophysiology*: Chronic bronchitis is a form of COPD characterized by an inflammation of the bronchi which stimulates the over-production of mucus causing frequent coughing. Chronic bronchitis is degenerative because over time, the persistent coughing causes increasing amounts of mucus to be produced which block the bronchioles and permanently damage the airways. Chronic bronchitis is defined as bronchitis lasting for three months or more in the year, over two consecutive years.

- *Causes and risk factors*: One of the main causes of chronic bronchitis is smoking but it can be caused by other irritants such as chemical vapours. Patients who experience recurrent respiratory infections are also at risk.

- *Symptoms*: These are generally the same as with acute bronchitis but chronic bronchitis is persistent and not self-limiting. Chronic bronchitis patients may develop the typical 'blue bloater' symptoms, because the skin appears blue around the lips (cyanosed) due to hypoxia (lack of oxygen) and is bloated due to fluid retention.

- *Diagnosis and treatment*: If the cough persists for more than three months in one year and the symptoms recur the following year, chronic bronchitis will usually be diagnosed based on the patient's history. Tests may be conducted to exclude other respiratory conditions (such as pneumonia or lung cancer). The best advice is to cease smoking (where applicable). Patients may be prescribed beta$_2$ agonists to stimulate bronchodilation and corticosteroids to reduce inflammation and ease breathing.

- *Complications*: Patients with chronic bronchitis are more at risk of other respiratory illnesses such as pneumonia or may develop respiratory acidosis (see Answer 8).

23 Cystic fibrosis **C. congenital**

- *Pathophysiology*: Cystic fibrosis (CF) is a congenital disease that affects the mucous glands and cells in the body, causing them to secrete excess mucus. These glands and cells are found in the respiratory, digestive and reproductive tracts. The excess mucus in the respiratory tract blocks the airways and causes frequent bacterial infections.

- *Causes*: It is caused by a faulty recessive gene that normally controls salt and water movement in and out of cells. When this gene is faulty, the cells and glands that normally secrete lubricating mucus, instead secrete excess salt (in the form of chloride ions) and not enough water, making mucus secretions thick and glue-like.

- *Risk factors*: There is no way of preventing CF if you have two copies of the recessive gene (see Figure 12.1). CF patients are at greater risk of recurrent respiratory infections. Families who are known to carry the gene can undergo genetic testing to determine if they are carriers.

- *Symptoms*: Patients have symptoms that affect a number of organ systems associated with the excess mucus that is secreted. Symptoms include recurrent respiratory infections, digestive problems and infertility.

- *Diagnosis and treatment*: Diagnosis is by screening. In the UK neonates are automatically screened as part of the heel prick test (which also screens for sickle cell anaemia and phenylketonuria (PKU)). There is no cure for CF and it is life-limiting (patients seldom survive beyond their mid-thirties). Treatment is focused on alleviating symptoms: for respiratory symptoms patients are prescribed bronchodilators and steroids to reduce inflammation and ease breathing. They may also be given an enzyme (DNase) to thin mucus. To relieve digestive symptoms, patients are given pancreatic enzymes to aid digestion along with vitamin and nutritional supplements. Daily physiotherapy is required to clear airways and help prevent respiratory tract infections. A lung transplant may be recommended if a patient suffers from respiratory failure and while this does not cure the disorder (because the defective gene is still present), it can relieve respiratory symptoms giving patients improved quality of life for a number of years.

- *Complications*: CF patients are at high risk of severe respiratory infections such as pneumonia. There is also a high risk of heart and lung failure.

24 Emphysema **D. degenerative**

- *Pathophysiology*: Emphysema is another form of COPD, it is a degenerative condition characterized by progressive shortness of breath due to chronic inflammation which damages the bronchioles and elasticity of the alveoli, impairing gas exchange. This damage is permanent and irreversible.

- *Causes*: The condition is caused by inhaled particles such as smoke or other irritants (such as hay or dust) which damage the alveolar membranes. Initially the lungs are able to compensate for the affected area using other areas of the lungs so that gas exchange remains efficient and no symptoms are noticed. However, as the condition progresses and the area of gas exchange is reduced, the patient will begin to experience symptoms (particularly upon exertion). In rare cases, emphysema is caused by a deficiency in the enzyme alpha 1-antitrypsin which damages the elasticity of the alveoli.

- *Risk factors*: Exposure to cigarette smoking is the biggest risk factor although certain occupations also carry a hazard, such as those that involve exposure to fumes or dust.

- *Symptoms*: Shortness of breath that gets progressively worse. This may be accompanied by a chronic cough and unintended weight loss as the patient expends more energy by breathing deeper to inhale sufficient oxygen. As the condition progresses, the patient may develop the characteristics of the 'pink puffer' – displaying a reddened complexion due to the effort required in breathing and hyperventilating in an attempt to inhale sufficient oxygen. They may also develop a characteristic expanded 'barrel chest' as the thoracic cage expands due to increased compliance in the lungs.

- *Diagnosis and treatment*: Like chronic bronchitis (another form of COPD), diagnosis is based on the patient's history. There will be a progressive deterioration in lung function tests (such as spirometer readings) and in ABG values. Further tests may be conducted to eliminate other possible respiratory disorders. The best advice is to cease smoking (where applicable). Patients may be prescribed beta$_2$ agonists to stimulate bronchodilation and corticosteroids to reduce inflammation and ease breathing.

- *Complications*: As with chronic bronchitis, emphysema patients are more at risk of other respiratory illnesses such as pneumonia or may develop respiratory acidosis (see Answer 8).

9 The digestive system

INTRODUCTION

The digestive system, consisting of the gastrointestinal (GI) tract and the accessory digestive organs, is responsible for processing all food and absorbing the nutrients derived from the diet into the blood to supply all the cells, tissues and organs of the body.

Diseases or disorders of any part of the GI tract can produce severe metabolic symptoms that can be life-threatening. An important part of diagnosis is to differentiate between the common disorders and the acutely life-threatening illnesses that often have similar symptoms.

Many of the diagnostic tools for investigative procedures on the GI tract are similar. The suspected location of ulcers or obstructions will determine the tool used. Sigmoidoscopy and colonoscopy can be used to visualize inside the lower regions of the GI tract along with a barium enema while a barium swallow is used to visualize the upper regions of the GI tract.

Several GI diseases can be prevented by eating a good diet that is low in salt and fat (particularly saturated fat) and high in fibre.

Nurses should know that the GI system is controlled by a range of nervous and hormonal messages and relies on an adequate supply of blood from the cardiovascular system. It is intimately related to these systems, therefore, a thorough understanding of these links is essential when diagnosing, treating and caring for patients with disorders of the GI system.

> ### Useful resources
>
> Nurses! Test Yourself in Anatomy and Physiology
>
> Chapter 9
>
> Ross and Wilson's Anatomy and Physiology in Health and Illness (11th edition)
>
> Chapter 12
>
> Symptoms, Diagnosis and Treatment
>
> Chapter 6

TRUE OR FALSE?

Are the following statements true or false?

1 The pyloric sphincter prevents the stomach contents from flowing back into the oesophagus.

2 Anorexia is a risk factor associated with cholecystitis.

3 Liver cirrhosis describes a group of chronic liver diseases.

4 Crohn's disease is a type of inflammatory bowel disease.

5 The most common cause of acute pancreatitis is obesity.

6 The bacteria *Helicobacter pylori* is the cause of 50 per cent of all peptic ulcers.

7 A common complication of repeated, acute hepatitis infections is development of chronic persistent hepatitis.

8 Colorectal cancer has a rapid onset and progression.

9 Lifestyle factors are strongly implicated as risk factors for colorectal cancer.

10 Antiemetic medication is usually prescribed to treat norovirus infections.

MULTIPLE CHOICE

Identify one correct answer for each of the following.

11 Cholecystitis is inflammation of which digestive organ?

a) stomach

b) liver

c) gall bladder

d) pancreas

12 Which of the following is not a symptom of Crohn's disease?

a) malaise

b) diarrhoea

c) weight gain

d) abdominal pain

13 Which of the following drugs is not used in treating Crohn's disease?

a) antidiarrhoea medication

b) corticosteroids

c) opioids

d) paracetamol

14 Symptoms of pancreatitis often start as an abdominal pain located in which region?

a) upper right quadrant

b) mid-epigastric region

c) lower left quadrant

d) lower back

15 The two major types of peptic ulcer are:

a) duodenal and stomach

b) oesophageal and stomach

c) duodenum and jejunum

d) stomach and jejunum

16 The main treatment for *Helicobacter pylori*-induced peptic ulcers is:

a) NSAIDs

b) antibiotics

c) antacids

d) paracetamol

17 Hepatitis describes inflammation of the liver most commonly caused by?

a) bacteria

b) fungus

c) protozoa

d) virus

18 Which of the following pre-existing conditions is not a risk factor for colorectal cancer?

a) Crohn's disease

b) colorectal polyps

c) liver cirrhosis

d) hereditary non-polyposis colorectal cancer

FILL IN THE BLANKS

Fill in the blanks in each statement using the options in this box.
Not all of them are required, so choose carefully!

gallstones	septicaemia
amylase	norovirus
appendicitis	endoscopy
ultrasound	faecal occult
influenza	atherosclerosis
ECG	

19 _____ infections are the most common cause of gastroenteritis.

20 An _____ scan is commonly used to diagnose cholecystitis.

21 _____ is a severe complication of cholecystitis that can be life-threatening.

22 A positive _____ _____ test for Crohn's disease will reveal blood in the stools.

23 Elevated _____ and lipase levels indicate pancreatitis.

24 The major diagnostic test for peptic ulcers is _____.

25 Increasing pain that tends to settle in the lower right side of the abdomen is a major symptom of _____.

ANSWERS

TRUE OR FALSE?

1 | **The pyloric sphincter prevents the stomach contents from flowing back into the oesophagus.**

The cardiac sphincter prevents the backflow of stomach contents into the oesophagus. If the sphincter mechanism fails, gastric reflux (heartburn) may arise (although this is not related to a cardiac problem). The cardiac sphincter relaxes during swallowing to allow food to enter the stomach. When this fails to occur, achalasia may develop. The main symptoms of achalasia are dysphagia (difficulty swallowing) and regurgitation of undigested food. A whole meal can become trapped in the oesophagus, resulting in severe chest pain which is often confused with heart pain. The pyloric sphincter controls the release of chyme into the duodenum from the stomach.

2 | **Anorexia is a risk factor associated with cholecystitis.**

Obesity and a high-cholesterol diet are risk factors for cholecystitis. Others include high oestrogen levels, diabetes mellitus, liver disease and pancreatitis. Symptoms of cholecystitis may develop quickly over a few hours, the main symptom being pain in the upper abdomen which is usually worse on the right side under the ribs. The pain may radiate to the back or right shoulder (see Figure 1.1). Patients may also develop nausea, vomiting, fever, indigestion and flatulence.

3 | **Liver cirrhosis describes a group of chronic liver diseases.**

Liver cirrhosis is characterized by irreversible destruction and scarring of the hepatic cells of the liver which are replaced by fibrous cells. Cirrhosis has many different causes, some of which are lifestyle-related, such as alcoholism and malnutrition. Other causes arise as complications of pre-existing diseases such as hepatitis or right-side heart failure which causes prolonged venous congestion in the liver. A liver biopsy will reveal the extent of liver tissue necrosis and fibrosis. A CT scan can also be used to determine liver size, abnormal masses or obstructions that may be present in the liver, affecting blood flow through the liver. Blood tests can determine if liver enzymes are elevated.

4 | **Crohn's disease is a type of inflammatory bowel disease.**

The severe inflammation can affect any part of the GI tract and can penetrate all layers of the intestinal wall, it may also involve lymph nodes. Ulcers may form when the inflammation progresses into the peritoneum.

5 **The most common cause of acute pancreatitis is obesity.**

Pancreatitis is inflammation of the pancreas. The most common cause of acute pancreatitis is alcohol abuse which accounts for the majority of cases in patients under 40 years. Gallstones are the second most common cause of acute pancreatitis, although this is more frequent in older patients. Other causes include tumours or cysts of the pancreas, kidney failure, drugs and metabolic or endocrine disorders such as high cholesterol or over-active thyroid. The main symptom of acute pancreatitis is a sudden onset of severe abdominal pain. Treatment involves supporting the body while it recovers by administering pain relief and supplying nutrients and fluids. With treatment, most patients recover in a few days but repeated episodes can lead to long-term inflammation (chronic pancreatitis). In around 20 per cent of patients, acute pancreatitis can become life-threatening. These patients are at risk of sudden hypotension, septicaemia and multi-organ failure.

6 **The bacteria *Helicobacter pylori* is the cause of 50 per cent of all peptic ulcers.**

The *Helicobacter pylori* (*H. pylori*) bacterium is the cause of 90 per cent of all peptic ulcers. Use of non-steroidal anti-inflammatory drugs (NSAIDs) (including low-dose aspirin for blood thinning) is another major risk factor. Other predisposing factors include genetic factors, stress or anxiety and blood type. Blood group A may predispose people to stomach ulcers while blood group O is associated with a predisposition to duodenal ulcers.

7 **A common complication of repeated, acute hepatitis infections is development of chronic persistent hepatitis.**

Recurrent episodes of acute hepatitis infections can prolong recovery by up to eight months in some patients who are then at risk of developing chronic active hepatitis. This is characterized by destruction of liver tissue, resulting in cirrhosis. In rare cases, patients can suffer from sudden and severe liver failure, which can be fatal.

8 **Colorectal cancer has a rapid onset and progression.**

Colorectal cancer has a long latent (asymptomatic) phase and progresses slowly remaining localized for a long time. Individuals are encouraged to report any persistent changes (six weeks or more) in bowel habit, such as diarrhoea or constipation or blood in the stools because early detection is key to successful treatment and recovery. Non-specific symptoms include abdominal pain, fatigue, bloating or unexplained weight loss.

9 **Lifestyle factors are strongly implicated as risk factors for colorectal cancer.**

A diet that is high-fat and low-fibre is a strong contributor to risk of colorectal cancer. This is because movement of digested food through the G I tract is slow in the absence of dietary fibre and moving slowly prolongs the mucosal lining's exposure to the faecal matter which may release toxins that encourage the cells to mutate. Faecal matter can also be irritating to the lining of the GI tract, causing unnecessary inflammation. Other risk factors include sedentary lifestyle, smoking, alcohol consumption and obesity.

10 **Antiemetic medication is usually prescribed to treat norovirus infections.**

Antiemetics are used to treat vomiting. However, gastroenteritis caused by norovirus infection is not normally treated with antiemetics because vomiting is the body's natural mechanism for expelling the virus (diarrhoea is another method). In severe cases, if a patient becomes severely dehydrated from repeated vomiting, an antiemetic may be recommended. Most patients do not seek medical attention in mild to moderate cases of gastroenteritis; patients are treated at home and advised to rest and drink plenty of water to prevent dehydration. Paracetamol can be taken to reduce fever symptoms. Patients should stay at home for 48 hours after they are symptom-free to prevent the spread of infection. If symptoms persist for more than three days or if the patient becomes severely dehydrated, medical attention should be sought. Children and older adults are particularly at risk of becoming dehydrated. Severely dehydrated patients may require hospital admission for IV fluids or a nasogastric tube to replace lost fluids. Although laboratory diagnosis is not normally necessary, norovirus can be diagnosed with a stool sample.

 MULTIPLE CHOICE

Correct answers identified in bold italics

11 **Cholecystitis is inflammation of which digestive organ?**

a) stomach   b) liver   *c) gall bladder*   d) pancreas

Cholecystitis is caused by the formation of gallstones (or calculi) which form when bile and cholesterol harden. Cholecystitis may be acute or chronic. Acute cholecystitis can be triggered by poor blood supply to the gall bladder, often when a gallstone lodges in the cystic duct, causing the gall bladder to become inflamed and painfully distended. Symptoms include sudden onset of severe right-side, upper-body pain which is constant and may be accompanied by nausea, vomiting or sweating.

12 **Which of the following is not a symptom of Crohn's disease?**

a) malaise   b) diarrhoea   *c) weight gain*   d) abdominal pain

Patients with Crohn's disease usually experience weight loss in addition to the other symptoms listed. Additional symptoms may include blood in the stools, nausea and vomiting. Abdominal pain is usually generalized but is sometimes localized to the lower right quadrant of the abdomen.

Crohn's disease is caused by a chronic inflammation of the lining of the GI tract – usually the ileum or colon. The cause is unknown although it is thought to be a combination of genetic and environmental factors.

13 **Which of the following drugs is not used in treating Crohn's disease?**

a) antidiarrhoea medication   b) corticosteroids   c) opioids
d) paracetamol

Along with drugs, treating Crohn's disease involves lifestyle changes and sometimes surgery. During acute attacks it is important to maintain fluid and electrolyte balance. Antidiarrhoea drugs (such as loperamide) are prescribed to relieve diarrhoea but are not recommended in patients with significant obstruction. Corticosteroids such as prednisone reduce inflammation, therefore relieving diarrhoea, pain and bleeding. Opioids may be prescribed to alleviate pain and diarrhoea. Around 80 per cent of patients will have surgery at some point to relieve symptoms or if the bowel becomes perforated or an acute obstruction develops. Surgery to remove the inflamed section of the GI tract relieves symptoms but it does not cure the disease – many patients report several years of remission from symptoms after surgery.

14 **Symptoms of pancreatitis often start as an abdominal pain located in which region?**

a) upper right quadrant   **b) mid-epigastric region**
c) lower left quadrant   d) lower back

In many patients the only initial symptom of pancreatitis is a pain in this region, centred on the navel, which is not relieved after vomiting. This pain may progress to swelling. In acute pancreatitis, the pain may be localized to the upper left quadrant and radiate to the back (see Figure 1.1). The pain often begins suddenly after eating a meal or drinking alcohol and is relieved when the patient is positioned on the knees and upper chest.

15 **The two major types of peptic ulcer are:**

a) duodenal and stomach   b) oesophageal and stomach
c) duodenum and jejunum   d) stomach and jejunum

Both of these types are chronic conditions that may be triggered by prolonged use of aspirin or another NSAID and excessive consumption of alcohol. Duodenal ulcers affect the upper part of the small intestine and account for about 80 per cent of peptic ulcers. Stomach (gastric) ulcers affect the mucosal lining of the stomach. Peptic ulcers are most accurately diagnosed by endoscopy, during which a sample may be taken to test for *H. pylori*, which can also be diagnosed by blood test (for *H. pylori* antibodies), stool antigen test or a urea breath test – elevated carbon dioxide (CO_2) isotope levels will be detected if *H. pylori* bacteria are present.

ANSWERS

The digestive system

16 **The main treatment for *Helicobacter pylori*-induced peptic ulcers is:**

a) NSAIDs   *b) antibiotics*   c) antacids   d) paracetamol

Treatment for *H. pylori* infection usually consists of a 1–2 week course of combination antibiotics along with a proton pump inhibitor (PPI) (such as omeprazole) or H_2-receptor antagonist (such as ranitidine) to reduce acid secretion in the stomach, giving ulcers time to heal. This is called eradication therapy. A combination of (usually three) antibiotics is used in case the bacteria have developed a resistance to antibiotics. The antibiotics normally used are: amoxicillin, clarithromycin, and metronidazole. These can cause unpleasant (but not normally harmful) side-effects such as nausea, vomiting or metallic taste in the mouth. Patients are tested after the treatment (usually using the urea breath test where CO_2 isotope levels on exhaled breath should be reduced if treatment is successful). Serious complications can develop from peptic ulcers, such as gastric bleeding, gastric obstruction and perforation of the stomach lining which can lead to peritonitis (inflammation of the abdominal lining).

17 **Hepatitis describes inflammation of the liver most commonly caused by?**

a) bacteria   b) fungus   c) protozoa   *d) virus*

Viral hepatitis is a common infection of the liver where tissue is destroyed by necrosis but in most patients the liver cells can regenerate with minimal permanent damage. There are five types of viral hepatitis: type A, B, C, D and E. They differ in their causes, severity and prognosis but all cause similar pathological changes to liver tissue. Hepatitis A is the most common form in the UK and often occurs in people who return from abroad because it is associated with poor sanitation and is caused by ingesting faecal matter (perhaps from contaminated fruit or vegetables). Many people now receive vaccination for hepatitis A before travelling to certain countries. Hepatitis B is transmitted through bodily fluids although a vaccine is widely available (and required for many health-care workers). Hepatitis C is also transmitted through body fluids but is mainly classified as a sexually-transmitted infection (STI), it is also associated with drug-users (because it can be transmitted through shared needles). There is no vaccine for Hepatitis C. The other forms of hepatitis are very rare in the UK.

18 **Which of the following pre-existing conditions is not a risk factor for colorectal cancer?**

a) Crohn's disease   b) colorectal polyps   *c) liver cirrhosis*
d) hereditary non-polyposis colorectal cancer

Crohn's disease and ulcerative colitis are bowel conditions that increase the risk of developing colorectal cancer because of the chronic inflammation of the lining of the GI tract. Colorectal polyps are strongly associated with a predisposition for colorectal cancer – the larger the polyp, the greater the risk. Hereditary non-polyposis colorectal cancer (HNPCC or Lynch syndrome) is a genetic disease associated with a very high risk of developing colorectal cancer as well as a number of other cancers of the digestive tract and patients should be offered regular screening.

FILL IN THE BLANKS

19 ***Norovirus*** **infections are the most common cause of gastroenteritis.**

The norovirus family of viruses is the most common cause of gastroenteritis in the UK. The norovirus infection is sometimes called the 'winter vomiting' disease. It is highly contagious and the virus can survive for several days in a contaminated area. It is spread through contact with an infected person, infected surfaces or objects, or by consuming contaminated food or water. Norovirus infections occur in all age-groups but are particularly common in contained environments such as schools, hospitals and nursing homes. Symptoms of a norovirus infection usually pass (without medical attention) within a few days and include nausea, vomiting, diarrhoea and in some cases a fever, headache, stomach cramps and aching limbs (see Answer 10).

20 **An** ***ultrasound*** **scan is commonly used to diagnose cholecystitis.**

Sound waves from the ultrasound scan will usually detect gallstones and ascertain also if the wall of the gall bladder is thickened (which occurs in cholecystitis). If the diagnosis is in doubt, then more detailed scans may be conducted. Treatment for cholecystitis often involves removal of the gall bladder to prevent recurrent episodes (which is common).

21 ***Septicaemia*** **is a severe complication of cholecystitis that can be life-threatening.**

If the gall bladder becomes severely infected or gangrenous, it can lead to septicaemia which can be life-threatening. Other possible complications include perforation of the gall bladder, or a fistula (channel) may form between the gall bladder and digestive tract due to prolonged inflammation.

22 **A positive** ***faecal occult*** **test for Crohn's disease will reveal blood in the stools.**

Other diagnostic tests for Crohn's disease may include X-ray of the small intestine which would indicate irregular mucosa and ulceration. A barium enema might indicate narrowing of the colon, while sigmoidoscopy and colonoscopy will identify patches of inflammation and also help eliminate ulcerative colitis.

23 **Elevated *amylase* and lipase levels indicate pancreatitis.**

Serum amylase and lipase levels will be grossly elevated in acute pancreatitis because the inflamed pancreas over-produces these two enzymes. Patients would be admitted to hospital for further tests and treatment. Further tests include ultrasound or a CT scan to detect an enlarged pancreas. If gallstones are suspected of causing acute pancreatitis, an endoscopic retrograde cholangio-pancreatography (ERCP) may be used to determine the exact location of the gallstone. There are no blood tests for chronic pancreatitis, although the physical state of the pancreas is assessed using the other tests described.

24 **The major diagnostic test for peptic ulcers is *endoscopy*.**

Upper GI endoscopy is used to confirm the presence of an ulcer. At the same time, tissue specimens or a biopsy may be taken to determine if ulcer is caused by *H. pylori* infection and to exclude GI cancer. A barium swallow may be used to diagnose upper GI ulcers when symptoms are not severe.

25 **Increasing pain that tends to settle in the lower right side of the abdomen is a major symptom of *appendicitis*.**

Appendicitis is an inflammation of the appendix, usually due to an infection or obstruction. The major symptom is pain in the abdomen that gets worse over several hours and tends to settle in the lower right side of the abdomen and gets worse when pressure is applied to the area. Appendicitis is considered a medical emergency, if left untreated the appendix can perforate which can cause life-threatening septicaemia. Appendicitis is usually treated by surgically removing the appendix (appendectomy). It is thought to occur more commonly in people who eat a low-fibre diet.

10 **The urinary system**

INTRODUCTION

The urinary (renal) system consists of the kidneys (that produce urine) and ureters, bladder and urethra (which store and transport urine before urination). The main function of this system is the filtration of blood and collection and excretion of waste products. Other vital roles of the kidneys include maintaining the acid–base balance of the blood; regulating intra-cellular and extra-cellular fluid balance; and maintenance of blood pressure.

   Disorders of the urinary system can be life-threatening if left untreated. Many of the symptoms of early disease are non-specific and include fatigue, lethargy, altered blood pressure, nausea and vomiting. Often it is only after certain blood tests, such as creatinine clearance levels, that renal problems become apparent. Specific symptoms include pain and change in frequency of urination. The location and nature of the pain usually indicate the source of the problem.

   It is important that such diagnostic tests are performed promptly and accurately interpreted so the necessary interventions can be made quickly as some renal disorders can deteriorate very quickly. Many disorders are associated with fluid imbalance and can be directly related to renal problems, or are secondary to a disorder of another organ system. These are commonly encountered by nurses in a variety of treatment settings therefore it is essential to have a thorough understanding of the urinary system and its associated functions.

Useful resources

Nurses! Test Yourself in Anatomy and Physiology

Chapter 10

Ross and Wilson's Anatomy and Physiology in Health and Illness (11th edition)

Chapter 13

Fluids and Electrolytes Made Incredibly Easy

TRUE OR FALSE?

Are the following statements true or false?

1 Irreversible destruction of renal tissue occurs in chronic kidney disease.

2 A pathophysiological sign of chronic kidney disease is an imbalance of fluids and electrolytes.

3 Acute renal failure occurs when there is a sudden interruption of renal function usually due to an obstruction.

4 Serum creatinine levels are a good diagnostic indicator of early acute renal failure.

5 Kidney stones develop when substances that normally dissolve in the urine form hard crystals.

6 Metabolic acidosis can occur due to excessive loss of bicarbonate ions from severe, prolonged diarrhoea.

7 Administering sodium chloride is the best treatment option for acute metabolic acidosis when blood pH is <7.1.

8 Cystitis is an infection of the upper urinary tract.

MULTIPLE CHOICE

Identify one correct answer for each of the following.

9 Chronic kidney disease occurs in how many stages?

   a) 2

   b) 3

   c) 4

   d) 5

10 Which of the following is not a classification of acute renal failure?

   a) prerenal failure

   b) interrenal failure

   c) intrarenal failure

   d) postrenal failure

11 Treatment of acute renal failure does not include which of the following?

   a) fluid restriction

   b) high calorie diet

   c) monitoring fluid and electrolyte balance

   d) administration of protein, sodium and potassium supplements

12 Which of the following is the most accurate measurement of the glomerular filtration rate?

   a) creatinine clearance

   b) blood pressure

   c) blood urea nitrogen

   d) urine output volume

13 Metabolic alkalosis is characterized by:

   a) a decrease in bicarbonate ions

   b) an increase in bicarbonate ions

   c) decreased blood pH

   d) an increase in hydrogen ions

14 Which of these situations is not a cause of metabolic acidosis?

   a) severe diarrhoea

   b) diabetic ketoacidosis

   c) excessive ingestion of alkali

   d) inefficient excretion of hydrogen ions

15 The main treatment for a lower urinary tract infection is:

   a) rest and fluids

   b) painkillers

   c) antibiotics

   d) IV fluids

16 Which of the following serum bicarbonate (HCO_3^-) values would indicate a patient is suffering from metabolic acidosis?

   a) < 26 mmol/L

   b) < 22 mmol/L

   c) > 22 mmol/L

   d) > 26 mmol/L

17 The most common form of treatment for larger kidney stones is:

   a) extracorporeal shock wave lithotripsy (ESWL)

   b) percutaneous nephrolithotomy (PCNL)

   c) ureteroscopy

   d) traditional surgery

18 Which of the following is not a symptom of glomerulonephritis?

a) kidney pain

b) frequent urination

c) haematuria

d) proteinuria

19 Which of the following is not advised in the treatment of glomerulonephritis?

a) drink plenty of water

b) limit salt intake

c) avoid alcohol

d) follow a strict diet

FILL IN THE BLANKS

Fill in the blanks in each statement using the options in this box.
Not all of them are required, so choose carefully!

compensation	1000 ml/minute
gallstones	septicaemia
amylase	dialysis
100 ml/minute	bicarbonate
sodium	creatinine
urea	renal colic
ECG	equilibrium

20 Clinical manifestation of acute renal failure is characterized by a sudden increase in serum _____ and _____.

21 Loss of _____ ions can cause metabolic acidosis in chronic kidney disease.

22 The severe pain of kidney stones is sometimes called _____ _____.

23 The normal creatinine clearance level is considered to be _____ or more.

24 To correct abnormal pH, metabolic acidosis may stimulate an opposing abnormality, respiratory alkalosis, this is known as _____.

25 _____is a treatment used in cases of kidney failure.

ANSWERS

 TRUE OR FALSE?

1 **Irreversible destruction of renal tissue occurs in chronic kidney disease.**

This is accompanied by gradual loss of kidney function. Occasionally, chronic kidney disease (CKD) arises suddenly, damaging the nephrons and resulting in a rapidly progressing disease that causes irreversible kidney damage.

2 **A pathophysiological sign of chronic kidney disease is an imbalance of fluids and electrolytes.**

Clinical features of fluid and electrolyte imbalance include hypervolaemia, hypocalcaemia, hyperkalaemia, hyperphosphataemia, hypertension, irregular heartbeat, fatigue and nausea. Patients with CKD will also experience symptoms such as fatigue, dyspnoea, haematuria, nocturia, itching, oedema and (in males) erectile dysfunction. Chronic kidney disease may develop as a complication of diabetes (types 1 and 2), hypertension and over-use of NSAIDs.

3 **Acute renal failure occurs when there is a sudden interruption of renal function usually due to an obstruction.**

Kidney obstruction is usually caused by renal calculi (stones). Other causes include hypovolaemia (low blood volume), poor circulation or kidney disease. It is a reversible condition but if left untreated, it can result in permanent damage and lead to CKD. During hypovolaemia, cells in the kidneys secrete renin that stimulates the production of angiotensin which causes blood vessels to constrict (vasoconstriction), resulting in increased blood pressure. Angiotensin also stimulates the secretion of aldosterone (vasopressin) from the adrenal cortex which causes the kidney tubules to increase the reabsorption of sodium and water into the blood. This increases the volume of fluid in the body, which also increases blood pressure.

4 **Serum creatinine levels are a good diagnostic indicator of early acute renal failure.**

Serum creatinine levels can remain within the normal range despite the loss of over 50 per cent of renal function, therefore this measurement is not a good diagnostic test in early stage acute renal failure.

5 | **Kidney stones develop when substances that normally dissolve in the urine form hard crystals.**

Also known as renal calculi, kidney stones develop when salts or minerals, normally found in urine, form solid crystals inside the kidney. Usually, these crystals are so small they pass harmlessly out of the body unnoticed. However, they can build up, forming a much larger stone that is difficult to pass, causing severe acute pain in the back or side (or occasionally the groin) which may last for minutes or hours. A small kidney stone (less than 4mm diameter) may be collected by filtering the urine though some gauze. For large stones (that will not pass) imaging techniques such as X-ray, CT scan or ultrasound can be used to locate the stone. Another imaging technique called intravenous pyelogram, IVP (or intravenous urogram (IVU)), is an X-ray of the urinary system using a contrast medium dye (injected into a vein) that highlights any blockages as the dye is filtered out of the blood by the kidneys. Once the stone is located, treatment and removal options can then be determined.

6 | **Metabolic acidosis can occur due to excessive loss of bicarbonate ions from severe, prolonged diarrhoea.**

Metabolic acidosis is an acid–base imbalance that occurs when the blood is too acidic. Acid is a by-product of the breakdown of fats during digestion. Normally the body can make bicarbonate ions to neutralize the acids produced in digestion but sometimes the body cannot make enough bicarbonate or too much of it is excreted. A lot of water and electrolytes (including bicarbonate) may be lost from the body during an episode of diarrhoea. It may also be caused by an accumulation of acidic hydrogen ions (H^+) caused by a respiratory disorder that prevents removal of excess CO_2 from the blood – respiratory acidosis (see Chapter 8, Answer 8).

7 | **Administering sodium chloride is the best treatment option for acute metabolic acidosis when blood pH is <7.1.**

Administering bicarbonate will neutralize the excess hydrogen ions, to treat acute metabolic acidosis. However, it is not normally recommended if the underlying cause of metabolic acidosis is unclear because this can lead to the opposite disorder – metabolic alkalosis. The kidneys help to regulate blood pH by excreting the hydrogen ions in urine and although this is slow, excretion in urine is the main way to eliminate excess acids from the body, especially in cases of mild metabolic acidosis.

8 | **Cystitis is an infection of the upper urinary tract.**

Cystitis is an infection of the bladder which is part of the lower urinary tract; the other part of the lower urinary tract is the urethra, an infection of which is called urethritis. A urinary tract infection (UTI) develops when part of the urinary tract becomes infected, usually by bacteria. Bacteria usually enter the urinary system through the urethra or, more rarely, through the bloodstream. UTIs are more common in females than males because the female urethra is shorter and closer to the anus than in males, which can allow bacteria from the anus to enter the urinary tract more easily. Symptoms include pain or a burning sensation during urination (dysuria), frequent need to urinate and lower abdominal pain. Infections are usually mild and usually resolve within 4–5 days. Antibiotics can be prescribed to clear the infection and speed up recovery. Some patients experience repeated UTIs, which can be treated with long-term antibiotics to prevent recurrent infections.

MULTIPLE CHOICE

Correct answers identified in bold italics

9 **Chronic kidney disease occurs in how many stages?**

a) 2   b) 3   c) 4   ***d) 5***

There are five stages of progression in CKD:

I.   Stage 1: Kidney damage with normal or increased GFR (≥ 90 ml/min).
II. Stage 2: Kidney damage with minor decrease in GFR (60–89 ml/min).
III. Stage 3: Moderate decrease in GFR (30–59 ml/min).
IV. Stage 4: Severe decrease in GFR (15–29 ml/min).
V.   Stage 5: Kidney failure (< 15ml/min or dialysis).

10 **Which of the following is not a classification of acute renal failure?**

a) prerenal failure   ***b) interrenal failure***   c) intrarenal failure
d) postrenal failure

This is not a classification of acute renal failure. Prerenal failure develops due to insufficient blood flow to the kidney (hypoperfusion) and may be caused by vasoconstriction, hypotension, hypovolaemia or decreased cardiac output. Prerenal failure can rapidly be reversed by restoring blood flow. Intrarenal failure occurs when damage occurs to the filtration mechanism of the kidney tubules. Postrenal failure is caused by obstruction of urine flow from the kidneys.

11 **Treatment of acute renal failure does not include which of the following?**

a) fluid restriction   b) high calorie diet   c) monitoring fluid and electrolyte balance   ***d) administration of protein, sodium and potassium supplements***

Intake of protein, sodium and potassium should be limited when treating for acute renal failure since levels of these may be elevated during the illness. All other measures should be taken when treating acute renal failure.

12 Which of the following is the most accurate measurement of the glomerular filtration rate?

a) creatinine clearance b) blood pressure c) blood urea nitrogen
d) urine output volume

Creatinine is filtered out the blood by the glomeruli and not reabsorbed by the tubules so it is an accurate measurement of the filtration rate of the glomeruli. It reflects how much fluid the kidneys have filtered over a 24-hour period. The test involves comparing the amount of creatinine in the blood with the amount excreted in urine over a given period. All urine produced over 24 hours is collected and a blood sample taken to test serum creatinine levels in the blood.

13 Metabolic alkalosis is characterized by:

a) a decrease in bicarbonate ions *b) an increase in bicarbonate ions* c) decreased blood pH d) an increase in hydrogen ions

In metabolic alkalosis, levels of bicarbonate ions in the blood serum will increase which in turn makes the blood more alkaline and increases the blood pH. This suppresses the respiratory centre in the medulla, inhibiting respiration. Levels of carbon dioxide in the blood will increase as the body attempts to correct the blood pH but this compensation by the respiratory system is usually limited. Metabolic alkalosis is the opposite acid–base disorder to metabolic acidosis.

14 Which of these situations is not a cause of metabolic acidosis?

a) severe diarrhoea b) diabetic ketoacidosis *c) excessive ingestion of alkali* d) inefficient excretion of hydrogen ions

Excessive alkali will increase the blood pH and so can trigger metabolic alkalosis but not metabolic acidosis. The other three situations can lead to development of metabolic acidosis.

15 The main treatment for a lower urinary tract infection is:

a) rest and fluids b) painkillers *c) antibiotics* d) IV fluids

Lower UTIs and mild-moderate upper UTIs are usually treated at home with a course of antibiotics for 3–7 days; the length of the course will depend on the severity of symptoms and the risk of developing complications. Painkillers such as paracetamol or ibuprofen may be taken to relieve pain (however, ibuprofen is not recommended during pregnancy). Treatment at home for an upper UTI usually involves taking antibiotics for 7–14 days. Some patients who develop upper UTIs will require hospital admission, namely, diabetics and patients who are immuno-compromised. Patients who develop severe upper UTIs and are over the age of 60 or pregnant may also require hospitalization. Hospitalized patients are treated with IV fluids and antibiotics and will have their blood and urine monitored regularly.

Patients usually respond well to hospital treatment and are discharged within seven days.

16 **Which of the following serum bicarbonate (HCO$_3^-$) values would indicate a patient is suffering from metabolic acidosis?**

a) < 26 mmol/L   *b) < 22 mmol/L*   c) > 22 mmol/L
d) > 26 mmol/L

The acceptable normal range of blood serum bicarbonate ions (HCO$_3^-$) is 22–26 mmol/L. When bicarbonate levels fall below 22 mmol/L, the patient is in metabolic acidosis. When bicarbonate levels in the systemic arterial blood exceed 26 mmol/L, the condition is called metabolic alkalosis.

17 **The most common form of treatment for larger kidney stones is:**

a) extracorporeal shock wave lithotripsy (ESWL)
b) percutaneous nephrolithotomy (PCNL)   c) ureteroscopy
d) traditional surgery

Larger stones (greater than 6mm diameter) and stones located in a ureter often require hospital treatment in the form of extracorporeal shock wave lithotripsy (ESWL), percutaneous nephrolithotomy (PCNL), ureteroscopy or traditional surgery. The treatment choice will depend on the size and location of the stone, although the most common method is ESWL which uses energy waves to break the stone into smaller pieces which then pass in the urine. ESWL is not suitable for obese patients; they usually undergo the surgical technique, PCNL. If the stone is in the ureter, ureteroscopy (also known as retrograde intrarenal surgery (RIRS)) may be recommended. Traditional surgery is only used in around 5 per cent of cases when no other method is suitable. If the stone is made up of uric acid, patients are advised to drink at least 3 litres of water every day to help dissolve the stone, however, this only works for this type of stone because they are much softer. Complications are rare with kidney stones, although until the blockage is removed patients are at increased risk of UTIs (see Answer 8). The most common complication is recurrence of the condition.

18 **Which of the following is not a symptom of glomerulonephritis?**

a) kidney pain   *b) frequent urination*   c) haematuria   d) proteinuria

Glomerulonephritis occurs when the glomeruli (tiny filters in the kidney) become inflamed. This may be due to a bacterial infection or can be secondary to a chronic autoimmune illness (such as SLE; see Chapter 2, Answer 17). When inflamed, the glomeruli do not filter the blood properly, causing an accumulation of salt and excess fluid. Severe glomerulonephritis may prevent urination for 2–3 days. Glomerulonephritis may not cause any obvious symptoms although small amounts of blood and/or protein may be present in the urine which may be apparent only upon testing. Not all patients experience kidney pain but when reported, it is important to exclude other conditions such as a UTI or kidney stones. In severe cases of glomerulonephritis, a noticeable amount of blood may be lost through the glomeruli, causing haematuria. If a large amount of protein is lost through the damaged glomeruli in the kidneys, the urine may be cloudy or frothy. The accumulation of fluid can lead to complications such as hypertension and in some cases, kidney disease or kidney failure can occur.

19 **Which of the following is not advised in the treatment of glomerulonephritis?**

a) drink plenty of water   b) limit salt intake   c) avoid alcohol
d) follow a strict diet

Patients are usually advised to restrict fluid intake and to avoid alcohol, their diet will have to be carefully controlled, usually under instruction from the GP or dietician, with advice about eating protein and controlling intake of potassium and salt. If the glomerulonephritis is caused by bacteria, an antibiotic will be prescribed and a corticosteroid may also be recommended. If the patient has high blood pressure, an angiotensin-converting enzyme (ACE) inhibitor may also be prescribed to reduce blood pressure and prevent further kidney damage and kidney failure. If the episode is secondary to another illness, it will need to be treated to prevent recurring episodes of glomerulonephritis.

FILL IN THE BLANKS

20 **Clinical manifestation of acute renal failure is characterized by a sudden increase in serum *urea* and *creatinine*.**

These are the first renal-related symptoms that appear in patients who have previously shown non-specific symptoms. The extent of elevated urea and creatinine levels will depend on the underlying cause and severity of the acute renal failure.

21 **Loss of *bicarbonate* ions can cause metabolic acidosis in chronic kidney disease.**

Metabolic acidosis is a symptom of CKD and can be diagnosed from arterial blood gas readings that will indicate a reduced blood pH below 7.35. When normal kidneys excrete excess hydrogen ions from the blood, the tubules reabsorb sodium and bicarbonate ions and return them to the blood. Metabolic acidosis develops because CKD limits excretion of hydrogen ions from the body. The excess hydrogen ions in cells cause the cells to secrete too many potassium, sodium and calcium ions, which causes an overall electrolyte imbalance.

22 **The severe pain of kidney stones is sometimes called *renal colic*.**

Renal colic is often used to describe the severe pain caused by a stone blocking a ureter. The severe pain is usually located on one or both sides of the back. It is described as sudden, excruciating spasms and is often accompanied with nausea, vomiting, fever, chills, sometimes the urine appears bloody or cloudy and the patient may experience frequent need to urinate or a burning sensation when urinating. Similar symptoms indicate a urinary tract infection so it is important to seek medical advice. Treatment of kidney stones depends on the type of stone: small stones often pass naturally in the urine; patients are usually advised to drink lots of water to encourage urination and keep the urine colourless. Often patients are asked to filter their urine through gauze so they will know when the stone has passed. Patients may be prescribed a painkiller and antiemetic to relieve symptoms. Pain usually subsides a few days after the stone passes.

23 **The normal creatinine clearance level is considered to be 100 ml/minute or more.**

A lower value indicates the kidneys are not functioning efficiently enough. Obese patients may not be able to obtain accurate creatinine clearance results. Creatinine clearance rates decrease with age. Blood urea nitrogen (BUN) levels are a measure of the amount of nitrogen in blood as determined by the amount of detectable urea. BUN is a useful indicator of renal function but creatinine clearance is considered more accurate.

24 **To correct abnormal pH, metabolic acidosis may stimulate an opposing abnormality, respiratory alkalosis, this is known as compensation.**

Compensation is triggered by the body to try to restore homeostasis of blood pH. There are two mechanisms: (1) respiratory hyperventilation; or (2) increasing bicarbonate production (by the kidneys). Hyperventilation can compensate for the decreasing blood pH by exhaling extra carbon dioxide; this raises the blood pH by removing the acid-causing carbon dioxide. Increasing the production of the alkaline bicarbonate compensates for metabolic acidosis by raising the blood pH, thus helping to neutralize the acidic nature of the blood.

25 **_Dialysis_ is a treatment used in cases of kidney failure.**

If the kidneys fail (such as in ESRF), an excess of waste products will accumulate in the blood. Dialysis is an artificial method of filtering the blood that mimics the normal functioning kidneys. Without dialysis treatment, kidney failure will be fatal. There are two types of dialysis: haemodialysis and peritoneal dialysis. Dialysis patients must observe a strict diet for their food and fluid intake. The only solution to long-term dialysis is a kidney transplant.

11 The male and female reproductive systems

INTRODUCTION

Reproduction is a complex process that demands the coordination of a series of anatomical and physiological events. The physiological and anatomical aspects of the reproductive tract are primarily associated with reproduction but there are also a number of psychosocial elements involved in the reproductive process. Dysfunction and disease of any of these components can cause acute and chronic illness, physical and emotional distress, fertility problems and sometimes even death.

While there are obvious differences in the structure and function of the male and female reproductive systems, a number of infectious diseases are common to both. Nevertheless, there are also a large number of conditions that are gender-specific and relate to the unique anatomy and physiology of the male and female reproductive systems. These are frequently a result of genetic, endocrine or structural abnormalities that affect reproductive function. Furthermore, a number of life-threatening malignancies are associated with specific reproductive organs.

Nurses should recognize that the male and female reproductive systems are susceptible to many disorders and that both genders are particularly vulnerable to sexually transmitted infections.

Useful resources

Nurses! Test Yourself in Anatomy and Physiology

Chapter 12

Ross and Wilson's Anatomy and Physiology in Health and Illness (11th edition)

Chapter 18

Symptoms, Diagnosis and Treatment

Chapter 5

Sexually transmitted diseases

http://www.cdc.gov/std

TRUE OR FALSE?

Are the following statements true or false?

1 Chlamydia infections may be asymptomatic.

2 The most common cause of pelvic inflammatory disease is the human papilloma virus.

3 Testicular cancer may be caused by significant trauma to the testes.

4 In many cases, prostate cancer will not shorten a man's natural lifespan.

5 The incidence of ovarian cancer in Western populations is declining.

6 Syphilis is a localized infection of the genitals.

7 Cryptorchidism is associated with an increased risk of testicular cancer.

MULTIPLE CHOICE

Identify one correct answer for each of the following.

8 Which of the following is not caused by pre-eclampsia?

a) hypertension

b) hypotension

c) proteinuria

d) oedema

9 The most common site of gonorrhoeal inflammation in males is:

a) the epididymis

b) the urethra

c) the testes

d) the prostate gland

10 The majority of breast tumours are described as:

a) malignant

b) ductal

c) benign

d) lobular

11 Which of the following is not a symptom associated with prostate cancer?

a) hypovolaemia

b) nocturia

c) haematuria

d) dysuria

FILL IN THE BLANKS

Fill in the blanks in each statement using the options in this box.
Not all of them are required, so choose carefully!

testicular	herpes simplex
human papilloma	ovarian
cervical	endometriosis
amenorrhoea	chlamydia

12   _____ cancer is linked to sexually transmitted infections.

13   Treatment of _____ may involve manipulation of the normal hormonal cycle.

14   _____ refers to absence of menstruation.

15   Genital warts are caused by the _____ _____ virus.

16   Prognosis for advanced _____ cancer is quite good.

ANSWERS

TRUE OR FALSE?

| 1 | **Chlamydia infections may be asymptomatic.**

Chlamydia is the most common bacterial infection transmitted through sexual contact. Incidence, particularly in young women, has risen dramatically over the past decade. Most females who have a chlamydia infection of the neck of the womb (cervicitis) have no symptoms (asymptomatic) and do not know that they are infected. In males, infection of the urethra (urethritis) is usually symptomatic, causing a white discharge from the penis with or without pain on urination (dysuria). Occasionally, the condition spreads to the upper genital tract in women (causing pelvic inflammatory disease) or to the epididymis in men (causing epididymitis). If untreated, chlamydia infections can lead to infertility.

| 2 | **The most common cause of pelvic inflammatory disease is the human papilloma virus.**

Pelvic inflammatory disease (PID) is an inflammation of the upper reproductive tract or pelvic cavity that may involve the uterus, the fallopian tubes, the ovaries and the pelvic peritoneum. It is caused by a bacterial infection and can develop if certain sexually transmitted infections (STIs), such as chlamydia or gonorrhoea, remain untreated. Certain procedures such as pelvic operation, postpartum infection, miscarriage or abortion may also increase the risk of developing PID. Individuals may be unaware of symptoms (silent PID) and even when symptoms are present, they can be vague, such as pain in the lower abdomen and pelvis, or deep pain experienced inside the pelvis during intercourse, bleeding between periods and after intercourse, unusual vaginal discharge, fever, vomiting and rectal pain. Most infections occur in sexually active women under 25 and incidence is increasing worldwide. PID has been identified as the leading cause of female infertility. It has also been associated with increasing the risk of ectopic pregnancy. Although the PID infection itself may be cured, effects of the infection may be permanent. This makes early identification essential to reduce the risk of long-term damage to the reproductive system. If the initial infection is mostly in the lower tract, fewer difficulties may be experienced after treatment. If the infection is in the fallopian tubes or ovaries, serious complications are more likely to occur. Treatment generally involves a combination of antibiotics since the infection may be due to multiple bacteria.

| 3 | **Testicular cancer may be caused by significant trauma to the testes.**

Testicular cancer is thought to be related to infection or trauma but there are also strong hereditary links. It mainly occurs in the 15–35-year-old age group and there has been a marked increased incidence in the past decade. Research now suggests that an undescended testicle at birth may be a risk factor for developing testicular cancer. It is the most common solid tumour in young males although it does occur in other age groups. For this reason, regular monthly testicular self-examination is recommended to check for an unusual hard mass. Treatment of testicular cancer using a combination of surgery, radiation therapy and in some cases chemotherapy has greatly increased prognosis. There can be psychosocial implications for patients who have treatment for testicular cancer related to altered body image or fertility problems.

4 **In many cases, prostate cancer will not shorten a man's natural lifespan.**

In many cases, prostate cancer will not affect a man's natural lifespan because it usually progresses very slowly – it can take up to 15 years for the cancer to metastasize (usually to the bones). The cause of prostate cancer remains unknown and the risk of developing the disease increases with age. In the early stages of disease, treatment can cure the cancer although, compared to other cancers, it does not respond well to treatment. Once it has metastasized to the bones, it cannot be cured and treatment is focused on prolonging life and relieving symptoms. Treatments include removing the prostate, hormone therapy and radiotherapy (using radiation to kill the cancerous cells). All the treatment options carry the risk of significant side effects including loss of libido, sexual dysfunction and urinary incontinence. For these reasons, many patients opt to delay treatment until there is a significant risk of metastasis.

5 **The incidence of ovarian cancer in Western populations is declining.**

The incidence of ovarian cancer is increasing in Western populations along with the number of deaths from the disease. Only 25 per cent of ovarian cancers are diagnosed in the early stages, when prognosis is most favourable. There are different types of ovarian cancer, which vary in severity. Genetic factors play a significant role in its development. Early indicators of the disease are vague but should be investigated when they persist. Symptoms are vague and include feeling bloated, indigestion, frequent urination, backache and constipation. The lack of a reliable screening test and non-specific symptoms of the cancer often delay early diagnosis. A large mass may be detected by pelvic examination. Transvaginal ultrasound is the current tool for diagnosis. Treatment involves surgery and chemotherapy, however, the outcome is very dependent on the stage of disease at time of diagnosis.

6 **Syphilis is a localized infection of the genitals.**

Syphilis is a systemic condition caused by the bacteria, *Treponema pallidum*. Transmission occurs upon contact with lesions (chancre) or body fluids during sexual contact. Characteristic symptoms of the early stages include painless chancre, malaise, a widespread systemic rash which may be present on the soles and palms. Loose necrotic tissue may also appear on the tongue. The next stage involves a period of latency which may persist for years. The final stage, tertiary syphilis, involves the appearance of necrotic and fibrosis tissue (gumma). These lesions may occur in bone, liver and the cardiovascular system. Neurosyphilis causes damage to the central nervous system resulting in dementia, blindness and motor disabilities. Some untreated patients never develop tertiary syphilis and rigorous treatment regimes have largely reduced the incidence of this stage. Congenital syphilis may cause considerable foetal abnormalities and is associated with significant *in utero* death. Treatment involves using long-acting penicillin or azithromycin for resistant strains.

7 | Cryptorchidism is associated with an increased risk of testicular cancer.

Cryptorchidism is a term describing incomplete testicular descent. Normally, the testes descends into the pelvis by the third month of gestation and then through the inguinal canal into the scrotum during the last two months of gestation, therefore premature baby boys have a greater risk of being born with undescended testes. Approximately 1 per cent of newborn boys have an undescended testis, a condition which usually resolves within the first year of life. Undescended testes are associated with increased risk of testicular cancer later in life and may lead to infertility. For these reasons, orchiopexy (surgical placement of testis in the scrotal sac) should be performed in cases of persistent cryptorchidism, preferably before two years of age, when degenerative tissue changes may begin to develop.

 # MULTIPLE CHOICE
Correct answers identified in bold italics

8 | Which of the following is not caused by pre-eclampsia?

a) hypertension **b) hypotension** c) proteinuria d) oedema

The causes of pre-eclampsia are not well understood but it is thought to be due to a problem with the blood vessels in the placenta that cause a disruption in the blood supply between mother and baby. The initial symptoms of pre-eclampsia are high blood pressure (hypertension), protein in the urine (proteinuria) and later oedema. If these symptoms develop, they are usually detected at routine antenatal check-ups. Pre-eclampsia can affect up to 10 per cent of first-time pregnancies although there is an increased risk if there is a family history or if it occurred in a previous pregnancy. Pre-eclampsia can only be treated by delivering the baby, so until that is possible (from week 37 onwards), patients will be monitored very closely during additional ante-natal appointments. In severe cases, the woman may be admitted to hospital. Patients are at risk of developing the more serious condition, eclampsia (convulsions) which can leave the mother permanently disabled or brain-damaged.

9 | **The most common site of gonorrhoeal inflammation in males is:**

a) the epididymis   **b) the urethra**   c) the testes
d) the prostate gland

The most common site of inflammation in males is the urethra which results in dysuria (painful urination) and a purulent (pus) urethral discharge. The bacteria attach to epithelial cells and damage the mucosa, causing an inflammatory response and formation of pus. Epididymitis may follow, although some males may remain asymptomatic. Gonorrhoea is caused by the bacteria *N. gonorrhoea*. Many strains of the bacteria have become resistant to treatment with penicillin and tetracycline making it more difficult to control but ceftriaxone and doxycycline-based therapies may be useful.

In females, the infection usually involves the endocervical canal and is frequently asymptomatic although it may also affect the accessory glands, causing more visible manifestations. PID usually develops as a serious complication. The newborn may become infected during birth, causing severe eye disease.

10 | **The majority of breast tumours are described as**

a) malignant   b) ductal   **c) benign**   d) lobular

Up to 90 per cent of tumours discovered in the breasts are benign. All breast lumps discovered by self-examination should be referred to the GP. A patient will probably be referred for a mammogram (X-ray of the breast tissue) although if the woman is under 35, this is unlikely because the breast tissue is more dense which makes the mammogram less reliable, these patients may be offered an ultrasound scan instead. A biopsy (usually a needle biopsy) may also be used to diagnose if the cells are malignant. Needle aspiration is used to treat benign cysts by draining fluid from the cyst. When breast tumours are diagnosed as malignant (after a biopsy) patients will usually be referred for further investigations, such as CT or MRI scans, to determine if the cancer has spread (metastasized). Although the earlier the diagnosis, the less likely the tumour is to have metastasized. Treatment and outcome will depend on the stage of the cancer.

11 | **Which of the following is not a symptom associated with prostate cancer?**

a) hypovolaemia   b) nocturia   c) haematuria   d) dysuria

Hypovolaemia describes low blood volume, typically due to a haemorrhage. It can lead to hypovolaemic shock which can be life-threatening. Prostate cancer does not normally cause any symptoms until the tumour is large enough to put pressure on the urethra. This results in problems associated with urination such as nocturia, dysuria and less frequently, haematuria. Symptoms of prostate cancer that is progressing include loss of appetite, weight loss and constant pain. Prostate cancer may be diagnosed from the screening test for prostate-specific antigen (PSA), which detects elevated levels of PSA in the blood. If PSA levels are raised, a digital rectal examination (DRE) will be performed to check for changes to the surface of the prostate gland. If prostate cancer is present, the gland may feel hard and bumpy rather than the normal smooth and firm textures. If there is a possibility that the cancer has metastasized, the patient will be referred for other diagnostic tests such as CT or MRI to evaluate the location and extent of metastases.

FILL IN THE BLANKS

12 *Cervical* **cancer is linked to sexually transmitted infections.**

Cervical cancer is strongly associated with sexually transmitted infections (STIs), particularly herpes simplex type 2 (HSV-2) and certain types of human papillomavirus (HPV). Vaccines against different strains of the virus have recently been developed and should prove effective in reducing the incidence of the malignancy. However, the vaccine is most effective in younger females who are not yet sexually active and so this population has been targeted in the vaccination programme. High risk factors for cervical cancer include multiple sexual partners, promiscuous partners, sexual contact at a young age and a history of STIs. Preliminary diagnosis via cervical smear is usually confirmed by biopsy, with surgery and radiation being the recommended treatment. The 5-year survival rate is 100 per cent with early diagnosis. Invasive forms of the disease have a less favourable prognosis and depend on the extent of metastasizes.

13 **Treatment of** *endometriosis* **may involve manipulation of the normal hormonal cycle.**

Endometriosis is a common condition in which small pieces of the uterine lining (endometrium) are found outside the uterus, such as in the fallopian tubes, ovaries, bladder, bowel, vagina or rectum. Endometriosis commonly causes pain in the lower abdomen, pelvis or lower back. It may also lead to fertility problems. However, some women have few or no symptoms. The cause of endometriosis is uncertain although it is thought to be hereditary. Treatments do not cure endometriosis but relieve the painful symptoms, either by pain medication, hormonal manipulation or surgery. Hormonal suppression aims to stop the growth of the endometrial tissue while ectopic endometrial tissue can be removed surgically. Depending on the age of the woman, a hysterectomy may be recommended.

14 *Amenorrhoea* **refers to absence of menstruation.**

Amenorrhoea describes the absence of menstruation and may be primary or secondary in nature. In the primary condition, the menarche (first menstrual period) has never occurred. This may be due to a genetic disorder, such as Turner syndrome (in which the ovaries do not function), or congenital defects that affect the hypothalamus or pituitary gland. A congenital absence of the uterus also causes amenorrhoea. Secondary amenorrhoea is the cessation of menstruation in an individual who has previously experienced cycles. It frequently results from hormonal imbalances when the hypothalamus may be suppressed by conditions such as sudden weight loss, eating disorders, or tumours. Systemic factors, such as anaemia or the administration of chemotherapy, may also be a cause of secondary amenorrhoea. Dysmenorrhoea refers to painful menstruation which may be due to the excessive release of prostaglandin during endometrial shedding.

15 Genital warts are caused by the *human papilloma* virus.

Genital warts are caused by an infection with the human papilloma virus (HPV) which is becoming more common. There are many types of HPV which affect the genital tract and some of these have been associated with cervical cancer (see Answer 12). The incubation period for HPV infection may be in excess of six months and the disease may be asymptomatic, depending on the location of the lesions. Pregnancy frequently promotes the growth and spread of this highly contagious disease. Genital warts may be removed by a number of different methods including surgery, laser, cryotherapy and topical caustic agents. However, in many cases they return.

The herpes virus is responsible for the occurrence of genital herpes characterized by the appearance of painful ulcerated vesicles (similar to those that appear on the mouth but not caused by the same strain of virus).

16 Prognosis for advanced *testicular* cancer is quite good.

The outlook for testicular cancer is very good because it is one of the most treatable types of cancer. Over 95 per cent of men diagnosed with early stage testicular cancer will be completely cured.

Even advanced testicular cancer, where the cancer has spread outside the testicles to nearby tissue, has an 80 per cent cure rate. Compared to other cancers, deaths from testicular cancer are rare. Treatment for testicular cancer includes the surgical removal of the affected testicle (which should not affect fertility or the ability to have sexual intercourse), chemotherapy and radiotherapy.

12 Genetics and hereditary disorders

INTRODUCTION

Genetics is the study of the inheritance of traits passed from parents to their children. Dominant genes will be expressed in any inheritance pattern while recessive genes will recede to the background – unless both parents carry the recessive gene. The expression of certain genes may also be influenced by environmental factors, for example, height is influenced by parental genes, health and nutrition.

For simple inheritance patterns, it is useful to draw a Punnett square to help understand and determine inheritance probabilities. This is used by genetic counsellors to calculate the likelihood of inheritance of particular traits.

Genetic disorders arise from changes (mutations) to genes or chromosomes and can also be affected by environmental influences. Disorders can be characterized as autosomal, sex-linked or multi-factorial.

Understanding genetics and inherited genetic disorders is an important aspect of healthcare in the twenty-first century. Many genetic disorders can be identified during pregnancy using screening tools such as amniocentesis or chorionic villus sampling (CVS). The ability to treat and empathize with patients and families affected by genetic and hereditary disorders is an important aspect of the care and support provided by health professionals.

Useful resources

Nurses! Test Yourself in Anatomy and Physiology

Chapter 13

Ross and Wilson's Anatomy and Physiology in Health and Illness (11th edition)

Chapter 17

Punnett square calculator

http://www.changbioscience.com/genetics/punnett.html

Haemophilia – the royal disease

http://www.sciencecases.org/hemo/hemo.asp

TRUE OR FALSE?

Are the following statements true or false?

1 Cystic fibrosis (CF) is an autosomal dominant disorder.

2 In autosomal recessive disorders, if both parents are affected with a disorder, their children will also have the condition.

3 Males are more likely to be affected by sex-linked recessive inherited disorders.

4 Physical signs of Down's syndrome are always detected at birth.

5 Primary treatment for cystic fibrosis involves managing symptoms.

6 Down's syndrome can be cured with gene therapy.

7 More than one form of haemophilia exists.

8 Haemophilia can remain undiagnosed into adulthood.

9 In Huntingdon's disease, behavioural symptoms often appear before neurological symptoms.

10 Development of some cancers involves the malfunction of certain genes.

MULTIPLE CHOICE

Identify one correct answer for each of the following.

11 If neither parent is affected but both are carriers of a gene for an autosomal recessive disorder, what percentage of children may be affected? *(Hint: it might help to draw a Punnett square.)*

a) 25%

b) 50%

c) 75%

d) 100%

12 In autosomal recessive disorders, if one parent is affected and the other is a carrier, what percentage chance will children have of being affected?

a) 25%

b) 50%

c) 75%

d) 100%

13 Which of the following is not a sex-linked disorder?

a) haemophilia

b) Klinefelter's syndrome

c) Turner syndrome

d) cystic fibrosis

14 In which of the following conditions will affected people have one unpaired X-chromosome?

a) haemophilia

b) Klinefelter's syndrome

c) Turner syndrome

d) cystic fibrosis

15 What type of essential molecule is mutated in cystic fibrosis sufferers, affecting transportation of chloride ions?

a) carbohydrate

b) amino acid

c) vitamin

d) lipid

16 How is Huntingdon's disease classified?

a) autosomal recessive

b) sex-linked

c) multi-factorial

d) autosomal dominant

17 Colour-blindness is classified as:

a) recessive, sex-linked

b) dominant, sex-linked

c) autosomal recessive

d) autosomal dominant

FILL IN THE BLANKS

Fill in the blanks in each statement using the options in this box.
Not all of them are required, so choose carefully!

Turner	Fragile X
multi-factorial	desmopressin
sex-linked	dominant
chromosomal	recessive
depression	antidiuretic hormone

18 Down's syndrome is a _____ disorder.

19 Excessive bleeding experienced by mild haemophilia A patients can be treated by administering the synthetic hormone _____ after injury.

20 Familial hypercholesterolaemia is a _____ inherited disorder.

21 Genetic disorders that are also influenced by environmental/lifestyle factors are called _____-_____ disorders.

22 Loss of personal independence can trigger _____ as a complication of Huntingdon's disease.

23 Phenylketonuria is an autosomal _____ disorder.

24 _____ _____ syndrome is an inherited learning disability mainly affecting males.

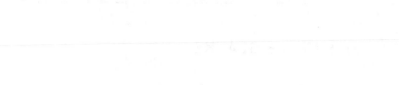

ANSWERS

TRUE OR FALSE?

1 **Cystic fibrosis (CF) is an autosomal dominant disorder.**

Cystic fibrosis (CF) is an autosomal recessive inherited disorder meaning neither parent suffers from CF but if they are *both* carriers of the CF gene, their children have a 25 per cent chance of being affected.

In autosomal dominant disorders, at least one parent is affected with the condition and their children will have a 50 per cent chance of being affected. Examples of autosomal dominant conditions include Huntingdon's disease and familial hypercholesterolaemia (FH).

2 **In autosomal recessive disorders, if both parents are affected with a disorder, their children will also have the condition.**

If both parents are affected, then all their children will definitely be affected with the disorder because there are no unaffected genes in the gene pool. Children can only inherit affected genes from both parents and so will suffer from the disorder.

3 **Males are more likely to be affected by sex-linked recessive inherited disorders.**

Some genetic disorders are caused by genes carried on the X-chromosome, these are known as 'sex-linked' ('X-linked') disorders. Males tend to be affected by recessive sex-linked disorders rather than females because males have only one X-chromosome while females have two. For females to be affected with a recessive sex-linked disorder, they need two copies of the affected gene, although this does not normally happen. Females with one recessive gene will not be affected but will be carriers. Examples of sex-linked disorders include haemophilia, Fragile X syndrome and Klinefelter's syndrome.

4 **Physical signs of Down's syndrome are always detected at birth.**

The physical signs of Down's syndrome include almond-shaped eyes, protruding tongue, flattened face, or small ears. Although the physical characteristics will be present at birth, they are not always detected, especially if the characteristics are not very pronounced. Nevertheless, the diagnosis is usually made shortly after birth. The baby may be born with other abnormalities such as congenital heart disease, cleft lip or palate, clubfoot or duodenal obstruction. Down's syndrome may be diagnosed before birth using chorionic villus sampling (CVS) (between weeks 10 and 13) or amniocentesis (between weeks 15 and 20) although both procedures carry an increased risk of miscarriage. A genetic karyotype (chromosome arrangement analysis) will confirm Down's syndrome by identifying the abnormality on chromosome 21. Alternatively, the quadruple screening test can identify pregnancies that are at greater risk of producing a Down's syndrome (or spina bifida) child, however, this test does not provide definitive diagnosis of these conditions.

5 | Primary treatment for cystic fibrosis involves managing symptoms.

Currently CF is incurable, therefore treatment focuses on maintaining quality of life. Treatments include salt supplements to correct electrolyte imbalance lost through sweat. Patients also take oral pancreatic enzymes to aid digestion since they may be deficient, or the enzymes may be unable to get to the necessary site of action due to the excess mucus in the GI tract. Antibiotics are often prescribed to treat respiratory infections which CF patients are prone to, due to the excess mucus in the respiratory tract. Physiotherapy is often performed several times a day on the chest to remove excess mucus. A mucus-thinning drug (DNase) can be administered which helps reduce infection and improve lung function. Heart and/or lung transplant is an option if required (after heart/lung failure). A lot of research is focused on developing gene therapy to replace the faulty gene in CF patients (see Chapter 8, Answer 23).

6 | Down's syndrome can be cured with gene therapy.

There is no cure for Down's syndrome. However, surgery and hormonal treatments are available to correct or alleviate some of the associated congenital disorders that often accompany the syndrome. Life expectancy is lower than normal and sufferers may have additional learning needs.

7 | More than one form of haemophilia exists.

There are two forms of the blood clotting disorder, haemophilia: haemophilia A and haemophilia B. The 'classic' form, haemophilia A, affects more that 80 per cent of all sufferers. It is caused by a deficiency or inefficiency of factor VIII, which is essential for blood clotting. The less common form, haemophilia B, is caused by a deficiency or inefficiency in clotting factor IX which is also involved in the blood clotting cascade.

8 | Haemophilia can remain undiagnosed into adulthood.

Depending on the severity of the disorder, patients may remain undiagnosed into adulthood. Such patients may not exhibit the characteristic excessive and spontaneous bleeding associated with haemophilia, but may complain of pain or swelling in weight-bearing joints such as hips, knees, ankles. These patients, classified as mild haemophiliacs, may report prolonged bleeding after surgery or dental extraction and may exhibit symptoms of internal bleeding or haematuria (blood in urine). Moderate and severe haemophiliacs are usually diagnosed earlier in life. Severe haemophiliacs may exhibit spontaneous bleeding and/or prolonged bleeding after minor trauma. Moderate haemophiliacs would also report excessive bleeding but may not experience regular spontaneous bleeding.

9 **In Huntingdon's disease, behavioural symptoms often appear before neurological symptoms.**

Behavioural symptoms are usually not specific and include hallucination, restlessness, paranoia, mood changes. Since this is an autosomal dominant disorder, people are usually aware of a family history and should seek medical advice as soon as symptoms arise. Neurological symptoms can be similar to those of Parkinson's disease (see Chapter 5, Answers 20, 27).

10 **Development of some cancers involves the malfunction of certain genes.**

All cancers develop from genetic mutations that cause uncontrolled cell growth. Mutations that affect cell growth can be caused by a number of factors either alone or in combination, namely, environmental factors such as exposure to radiation or certain chemicals (benzene). The mutation may occur sporadically or the faulty gene may be inherited but mutates further upon exposure to environmental carcinogens. Inherited mutations in some genes are known to pose an increased risk of certain cancers. Examples include BRCA1/2 mutations which are strongly associated with an increased risk of breast and/or ovarian cancers, or Lynch syndrome (HNPCC) an autosomal dominant condition that carries a very high risk of colon cancer at an early age.

 MULTIPLE CHOICE

Correct answers identified in bold italics

11 **If neither parent is affected but both are carriers of a gene for an autosomal recessive disorder, what percentage of children may be affected?**

a) 25%   b) 50%   c) 75%   d) 100%

Children of two heterozygous parents have a one in four chance of being affected (Figure 12.1 – option (4)) with an autosomal recessive disorder (such as cystic fibrosis or phenylketonuria (PKU)) and a 50 per cent chance of being carriers (Figure 12.1 – options (2), (3)). When one parent is affected but the other is not a carrier (that is, homozygous dominant), no children will be affected with the disorder but will all be carriers (Figure 12.2).

Figure 12.1 **Punnett square for cystic fibrosis** (both parents carriers)

Male parent (carrier) ♀ ♂ Female parent (carrier)	C	c̄
C	(1) CC	(2) Cc̄
c̄	(3) Cc̄	(4) c̄c̄

C = dominant, healthy allele
c̄ = recessive allele associated with CF

Figure 12.2 **Punnett square for phenylketonuria inheritance** (father not carrier)

Male parent (not carrier) ♀ ♂ Female parent (affected)	P	P
p̄	(1) Pp̄	(2) Pp̄
p̄	(3) Pp̄	(4) Pp̄

P = dominant, healthy allele
p̄ = recessive allele associated with phenylketonuria

12 **In autosomal recessive disorders, if one parent is affected and the other is a carrier, what percentage chance will children have of being affected?**

a) 25%   *b)* **50%**   c) 75%   d) 100%

Each child will have a one in two (50 per cent) chance of being affected with the disorder (Figure 12.3 – options (2), (4)) and a one in two (50 per cent) chance of being a carrier of the disorder (Figure 12.3 – options (1), (3)).

Figure 12.3 Punnett square for autosomal recessive inheritance
(father carrier)

♀ Female parent (affected) \ ♂ Male parent (carrier)	P	p̄
p̄	(1) Pp̄	(2) p̄p̄
p̄	(3) Pp̄	(4) p̄p̄

P = dominant, healthy allele
p̄ = recessive allele associated with disorder

13 **Which of the following is not a sex-linked disorder?**

a) haemophilia   b) Klinefelter's syndrome   c) Turner syndrome
d) cystic fibrosis

All these conditions are genetic disorders. However, cystic fibrosis is not a sex-linked condition because it is carried on chromosome 7. All the other conditions are inherited through the X-chromosome. Haemophilia is a blood-clotting disorder. Affected people bleed profusely because they are lacking a clotting factor that controls coagulation (see Answers 7, 8). Klinefelter's syndrome is a trisomy condition in males (who have an extra

X-chromosome and so have 47 chromosomes), with the sex chromosomes having an XXY arrangement. Turner syndrome is a monosomy sex-linked disorder that affects females. Such patients have only one unpaired X-chromosome, therefore, they fail to develop and mature as normal females.

14 **In which of the following conditions will affected people have one unpaired X-chromosome?**

a) haemophilia   b) Klinefelter's syndrome   *c) Turner syndrome*
d) cystic fibrosis

Turner syndrome is an unusual sex-linked disorder because it affects females. Affected women are missing an X-chromosome so it is a monosomy condition with only 45 chromosomes in total. Characteristic physical abnormalities include short stature, swelling, broad chest, low hairline, low-set ears and webbed necks. Patients with Turner syndrome typically have non-functioning ovaries, which results in amenorrhoea (absence of menstrual cycle) and sterility (see Chapter 11, Answer 14). Approximately 98 per cent of foetuses with Turner syndrome are lost through spontaneous miscarriage.

15 **What type of essential molecule is mutated in cystic fibrosis sufferers, affecting transportation of chloride ions?**

a) carbohydrate   *b) amino acid*   c) vitamin   d) lipid

Sufferers of cystic fibrosis have an abnormal protein, phenylalanine, due to the absence of an essential amino acid, that affects the movement of chloride ions across cell membranes. The lack of this amino acid leads to the formation of thick, sticky mucus in the lungs, digestive tract and other parts of the body. This mucus causes respiratory, metabolic and fertility problems in sufferers and it can often become infected, leaving patients susceptible to frequent respiratory infections (see Chapter 8, Answer 23).

16 **How is Huntingdon's disease classified?**

a) autosomal recessive   b) sex-linked   c) multi-factorial
d) autosomal dominant

Huntingdon's disease is an inherited neurodegenerative disease caused by a defect on chromosome 4. It is an autosomal dominant disease because when one parent has Huntington's disease, children will have at least a 50 per cent chance of being sufferers (Figure 12.4). If both parents are affected by the gene, their children have a 75 per cent chance of developing the disease (Figure 12.5 – options (1), (2), (3)). It is extremely rare for the affected parent to be homozygous for the dominant gene (has two affected alleles as in Figure 12.5 – option (1)), in this case, all children will have the dominant gene and therefore will develop the condition.

Figure 12.4 Punnett square for inheritance of Huntingdon's disease
(mother unaffected)

♀ Female parent (unaffected) \ ♂ Male parent (affected)	H	h
h	(1) Hh	(2) hh
h	(3) Hh	(4) hh

H = dominant, disease-causing allele
h = recessive, normal allele

Figure 12.5 Punnett square for inheritance of Huntingdon's disease
(both parents affected)

♀ Female parent (affected) \ ♂ Male parent (affected)	H	h
H	(1) HH	(2) Hh
h	(3) Hh	(4) hh

H = dominant, disease-causing allele
h = recessive, normal allele

17 **Colour-blindness is classified as:**

a) recessive, sex-linked   b) dominant, sex-linked
c) autosomal recessive   d) autosomal dominant

Colour-blindness (colour vision deficiency) is a recessive trait which affects the function of cells in the retina of the eye that detect colours and therefore reduces the ability of the affected individual to interpret colours. Most of the genes involved in colour vision are transmitted on the X-chromosome, therefore, it is a recessive, sex-linked condition that mainly affects males. A colour-blind male will pass his recessive gene for the condition to all female children who will carry the recessive gene (Figure 12.6 – options (1), (3)). The sons of a female carrier have a 50 per cent chance of being affected. (Figure 12.7 – option (4)). The most common form of the disorder (about 95 per cent) is red–green colour-blindness where sufferers cannot distinguish between red and green. Less than 5 per cent of sufferers cannot distinguish between blue and yellow, while the rarest form of the disorder is 'true' colour-blindness when no colours are detected and everything is interpreted as black, white and shades of grey (these patients have poor vision and are very light-sensitive). Diagnosis is usually via a series of tests involving coloured dots and although there is no cure, most sufferers adapt very well and lead normal lives (red–green colour blind people are permitted to drive in most countries).

Figure 12.6 Punnett square for sex-linked inheritance of colour-blindness (father affected, mother carrier)

♀ Female parent (carrier) ╲ ♂ Male parent (affected)	X$\bar{c}$	Y
XC	(1) XC X$\bar{c}$	(2) XC Y
X$\bar{c}$	(3) X$\bar{c}$ X$\bar{c}$	(4) X$\bar{c}$ Y

XC = dominant allele for normal colour vision carried on X-chromosome
X$\bar{c}$ = recessive allele for colour-blindness, carried on X-chromosome
Y = normal Y (male) chromosome that carries no gene for colour vision

Figure 12.7 Punnett square for sex-linked inheritance of colour-blindness (mother carrier)

	XC	Y
Male parent (unaffected) ♂ / **Female parent** (carrier) ♀		
XC	(1) XC XC	(2) XC Y
X$\bar{c}$	(3) XC X$\bar{c}$	(4) X$\bar{c}$ Y

XC = dominant allele for normal colour vision carried on X-chromosome
X$\bar{c}$ = recessive allele for colour-blindness, carried on X-chromosome
Y = normal Y (male) chromosome that carries no gene for colour vision

FILL IN THE BLANKS

18 **Down's syndrome is a *chromosomal* disorder.**

Also called Trisomy 21, Down's syndrome is caused by an extra chromosome 21 which means people with the condition have a total of 47 chromosomes (instead of 46). It is strongly associated with the age of the mother, being more common in children born to mothers over 35 years. This is thought to be caused by changes to the ova as the woman ages.

19 **Excessive bleeding experienced by mild haemophilia A patients can be treated by administering the synthetic hormone *desmopressin* after injury.**

Desmopressin is usually administered intravenously and works by stimulating the production of clotting factor VIII. It can produce side effects including headache and nausea. Desmopressin is not as effective at treating mild haemophilia B because this form is caused by a lack of clotting factor IX. Haemophilia B can be treated with the drug nonacog alfan. Moderate and severe haemophiliacs will be treated prophylactically.

20 | Familial hypercholesterolaemia is a _dominant_ inherited disorder.

Familial hypercholesterolaemia (FH) is characterized by high levels of low-density lipoprotein (LDL) cholesterol in the blood which leaves patients at greater risk of developing cardiovascular diseases at a younger age. Since it is a dominant inherited disorder, it is quite common, occurring in around one in five hundred people. Children of infected people have a 50 per cent chance of being affected. Affected individuals will have elevated serum cholesterol readings and should have their levels monitored regularly. These patients are usually prescribed statins to help reduce the levels of LDL in the blood by reducing the amount of cholesterol naturally produced by the liver. Patients are also encouraged to make lifestyle adjustments to reduce their risk of developing cardiovascular diseases.

21 | Genetic disorders that are also influenced by environmental/ lifestyle factors are called _multi-factorial_ disorders.

One example of a multi-factorial disorder is a cleft lip or a cleft palate. Multi-factorial genetic disorders can be very complex. Along with genetic factors, there are lifestyle factors that can contribute to these conditions, such as maternal smoking and alcohol consumption as well as maternal obesity and lack of folic acid in the diet during early pregnancy. Cleft conditions are usually treated successfully with surgery and sometimes require speech therapy. Neural tube defects (spina bifida) are also considered multi-factorial disorders and are associated with diets low in folic acid.

22 | Loss of personal independence can trigger _depression_ as a complication of Huntingdon's disease.

As the disease progresses, patients will need assistance and supervision, eventually requiring 24-hour care. This loss of independence can lead to depression in patients. Patients often report having witnessed the devastating effects on a family member who previously suffered with the disease. Knowledge of how devastating the disease is can be a major cause of depression and even suicide. Depression is a common problem among sufferers of genetic and inherited disorders, particularly in patients who lack personal independence.

23 | Phenylketonuria is an autosomal _recessive_ disorder.

Phenylketonuria (PKU) is an inherited recessive disorder (see Figures 12.2 and 12.3) that develops when the body cannot synthesize the enzyme required to convert the amino-acid phenylalanine to tyrosine. This conversion is necessary to prevent an accumulation of phenylalanine in the body since it is toxic in large amounts, causing irreversible damage to many organs. There is no cure for PKU although all newborns in the UK are screened for the disorder (during the heel-prick test); treatment is mainly dietary where sufferers who adhere to a strict diet (limiting phenylalanine intake) can lead relatively normal lives.

24   ***Fragile X*** **syndrome is an inherited learning disability mainly affecting males.**

Fragile X syndrome is a dominant sex-linked disorder that causes a spectrum of characteristic physical, intellectual, emotional and behavioural features which range from severe to mild. It accounts for the majority of learning disabilities affecting males. Physical symptoms include long face, large ears and flat feet. A range of emotional and behavioural symptoms will be present which include shyness, inability to make eye contact and obsessive behaviours. Some individuals with Fragile X syndrome also meet the diagnostic criteria for autistic spectrum disorders (ASDs). Although rare in females, those who have the syndrome experience symptoms to a lesser degree because of their second X-chromosome. Fragile X syndrome can be diagnosed during pregnancy by amniocentesis. There is no cure for the condition and affected individuals are recommended for educational and behavioural therapies.

Glossary

Aetiology: the study of causes of disease.

Apoptosis: a normal part of cell development when the cell undergoes programmed cell death through a series of biochemical changes in the cell. The cell debris from apoptosis does not cause harm to the adjacent cells; this is how it differs from necrosis.

Bradycardia: slow heart beat (usually less than 60 beats per minute in a resting adult).

Bradykinesia: slowness of movement.

Cardiac arrhythmia: abnormal electrical activity in the heart. The heart beat may be too fast or too slow and may be regular or irregular.

Cyanosis: blue/purple discoloration of the skin and mucous membranes, characteristic of hypoxia.

Dysaesthesia: numbness or tingling ('pins and needles').

Dysphagia: difficulty swallowing.

Dyspnoea: shortness of breath (SOB), breathlessness.

Dysuria: painful urination.

Fatigue: tiredness, weariness.

Glycosuria: (or glucosuria) glucose in the urine.

Gram's stain: a staining technique used to classify bacteria. Gram-positive bacteria retain the violet stain; gram-negative bacteria do not.

Haematuria: blood in urine, usually arising from the kidneys.

Haemodilution: increase in plasma volume in the blood, which consequently dilutes the concentration of red blood cells.

Hypercalcaemia: elevated calcium levels in the blood.

Hypercapnia: increased concentration of carbon dioxide in the blood.

Hyperglycaemia: excessively high blood glucose levels (indicates uncontrolled diabetes).

Hyperkalaemia: high potassium levels in the blood.

Hypermagnesaemia: high levels of magnesium in the blood (can occur in renal failure when patients are given excess laxatives or antacids, can also be caused by enemas).

Hyperphosphataemia: elevated levels of phosphate in the blood (common in chronic kidney disease).

Hypersecretion: excess secretion.

Hypertension: high blood pressure (usually describes *persistent* high blood pressure).

Hyperthermia: excessively high core body temperature (usually caused by sunstroke or overwhelming bacterial infection).

Hyperthyroidism: overactive thyroid, secreting excess thyroid hormones.

Hyperventilate: over-breathing; when breathing is faster and deeper than necessary (causing excessive carbon dioxide to be exhaled).

Hypervolaemia: (or fluid overload) abnormally increased volume of blood (most commonly due to congestive heart failure).

Hypocalcaemia: low serum calcium levels (possibly due to vitamin D deficiency).

Hypocapnia: abnormally low levels of carbon dioxide in the blood.

Hypoglycaemia: low blood glucose (sugar) levels (possibly due to administration or secretion of too much insulin).

Hypokalaemia: low potassium levels in the blood, can be caused by diuretics and laxatives.

Hypomagnesaemia: low levels of magnesium in the blood (often refers to systemic magnesium deficiency, can be caused by chronic diarrhoea or alcoholism).

Hypoperfusion: decreased blood flow through an organ or tissue.

Hypophosphataemia: abnormally low levels of phosphate in the blood (common in malnutrition).

Hyposecretion: decrease in secretion or release of a substance.

Hypotension: abnormally low blood pressure.

Hypothermia: excessively low core body temperature.

Hypothyroidism: under-active thyroid, secreting insufficient thyroxine.

Hypovolaemia: decreased volume of circulating blood (specifically blood plasma), may be due to dehydration, haemorrhage, excessive diarrhoea or diuretic drugs.

Hypoxia: lack of oxygen.

Ischaemia: decreased blood supply to organ or tissue.

Lethargy: tiredness, sluggish.

Metastasis: movement of malignant cells from one location in the body to another, usually via the blood or lymphatic system.

Necrosis: an undesirable form of cell death usually caused by factors external to the cell, such as trauma, toxins or infection. Gangrene is an example of a dangerous accumulation of necrotic tissue.

Nocturia: frequent urination at night.

Pallor: pale in colour.

Palpate: examination of the body by touching or pressing with the fingers or the palm of the hand.

Palpitation: excessive beating of the heart.

Pathogen: disease-causing agent or microorganism.

Pathophysiology: changes to the normal anatomy and physiology due to illness or disease.

Polydipsia: excessive thirst.

Polyphagia: increased appetite.

Polyuria: excessive urination.

Post-prandial: after eating.

Pre-prandial: before eating.

Proteinuria: protein in the urine.

Reperfusion: restoration of blood flow to an organ or tissue (for example, after MI or CVA).

Resistance: opposition to airflow in the lungs or chest wall.

Septicaemia: blood poisoning, sepsis, septic shock.

Tachycardia: rapid heartbeat (usually more than 100 beats per minute in a resting adult).

Urticaria: hives.

Vasoconstriction: narrowing of blood vessels due to contraction of smooth muscle surrounding the walls, reduces blood flow (commonly caused by increased calcium concentration in cells).

Vasodilation: widening of blood vessels due to relaxation of smooth muscle surrounding the walls, increases blood flow (decrease in blood pressure).

LIBRARY, UNIVERSITY OF CHESTER

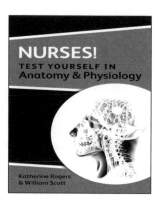

NURSES! TEST YOURSELF IN ANATOMY & PHYSIOLOGY

Katherine Rogers and William Scott

9780335241637 (Paperback)
April 2011

eBook also available

Looking for a quick and effective way to revise and test your knowledge? This handy book is the essential self-test resource for nurses studying basic anatomy & physiology and preparing for exams. This book includes over 450 questions in total, each with fully explained answers.

Key features:

- Organised into body systems chapters
- Includes a range of question types
- Provides a list of clearly explained answers to questions

www.openup.co.uk

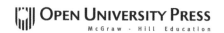 OPEN UNIVERSITY PRESS
McGraw - Hill Education